DATE DUE

DEC 1 0 2008	
FEB 2 5 2009	
APR 2 2 2009	
APR 0 5 2010	
DEC 2 0 2010	
DEC 1 7 2012	

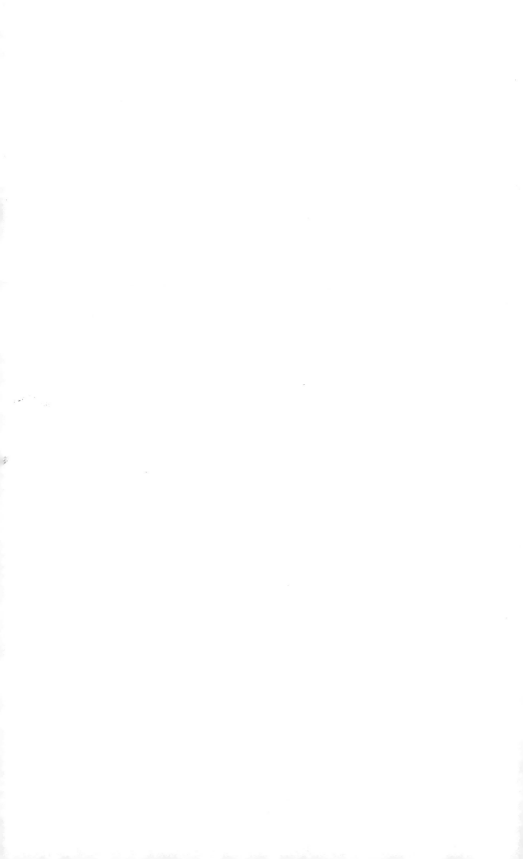

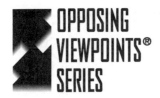
OPPOSING VIEWPOINTS® SERIES

Alternative Medicine

Other Books of Related Interest:

Opposing Viewpoints Series
Conserving the Environment
Medicine

At Issue Series
Are Americans Overmedicated?

Current Controversies Series
Healthcare

"Congress shall make no law ... abridging the freedom of speech, or of the press."

First Amendment to the U.S. Constitution

The basic foundation of our democracy is the First Amendment guarantee of freedom of expression. The Opposing Viewpoints series is dedicated to the concept of this basic freedom and the idea that it is more important to practice it than to enshrine it.

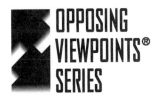

OPPOSING VIEWPOINTS® SERIES

Alternative Medicine

David M. Haugen, Book Editor

GREENHAVEN PRESS

An imprint of Thomson Gale, a part of The Thomson Corporation

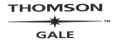

THOMSON
*
™
GALE

Detroit • New York • San Francisco • New Haven, Conn. • Waterville, Maine • London

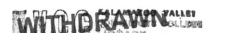

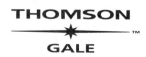

Christine Nasso, *Publisher*
Elizabeth Des Chenes, *Managing Editor*

© 2008 The Gale Group.

Star logo is a trademark and Gale and Greenhaven Press are registered trademarks used herein under license.

For more information, contact:
Greenhaven Press
27500 Drake Rd.
Farmington Hills, MI 48331-3535
Or you can visit our Internet site at http://www.gale.com

Cover photograph reproduced by permission of photos.com.

ISBN-13: 978-0-7377-3820-9 (hardcover)
ISBN-10: 0-7377-3820-0
ISBN-13: 978-0-7377-3821-6 (pbk.)
ISBN-10: 0-7377-3821-9

2007935072

Contents

Chapter 3: Can Alternative and Conventional Medicine Work Together?

Chapter 4: What Should Government Do to Research and Regulate Alternative Medicine?

Why Consider Opposing Viewpoints?

> *"The only way in which a human being can make some approach to knowing the whole of a subject is by hearing what can be said about it by persons of every variety of opinion and studying all modes in which it can be looked at by every character of mind. No wise man ever acquired his wisdom in any mode but this."*
>
> *John Stuart Mill*

In our media-intensive culture it is not difficult to find differing opinions. Thousands of newspapers and magazines and dozens of radio and television talk shows resound with differing points of view. The difficulty lies in deciding which opinion to agree with and which "experts" seem the most credible. The more inundated we become with differing opinions and claims, the more essential it is to hone critical reading and thinking skills to evaluate these ideas. Opposing Viewpoints books address this problem directly by presenting stimulating debates that can be used to enhance and teach these skills. The varied opinions contained in each book examine many different aspects of a single issue. While examining these conveniently edited opposing views, readers can develop critical thinking skills such as the ability to compare and contrast authors' credibility, facts, argumentation styles, use of persuasive techniques, and other stylistic tools. In short, the Opposing Viewpoints series is an ideal way to attain the higher-level thinking and reading skills so essential in a culture of diverse and contradictory opinions.

In addition to providing a tool for critical thinking, Opposing Viewpoints books challenge readers to question their own strongly held opinions and assumptions. Most people form their opinions on the basis of upbringing, peer pressure, and personal, cultural, or professional bias. By reading carefully balanced opposing views, readers must directly confront new ideas as well as the opinions of those with whom they disagree. This is not to simplistically argue that everyone who reads opposing views will—or should—change his or her opinion. Instead, the series enhances readers' understanding of their own views by encouraging confrontation with opposing ideas. Careful examination of others' views can lead to the readers' understanding of the logical inconsistencies in their own opinions, perspective on why they hold an opinion, and the consideration of the possibility that their opinion requires further evaluation.

Evaluating Other Opinions

To ensure that this type of examination occurs, Opposing Viewpoints books present all types of opinions. Prominent spokespeople on different sides of each issue as well as well-known professionals from many disciplines challenge the reader. An additional goal of the series is to provide a forum for other, less-known, or even unpopular viewpoints. The opinion of an ordinary person who has had to make the decision to cut off life support from a terminally ill relative, for example, may be just as valuable and provide just as much insight as a medical ethicist's professional opinion. The editors have two additional purposes in including these less-known views. One, the editors encourage readers to respect others' opinions—even when not enhanced by professional credibility. It is only by reading or listening to and objectively evaluating others' ideas that one can determine whether they are worthy of consideration. Two, the inclusion of such viewpoints encourages the important critical thinking skill of objectively evaluating an author's credentials and bias. This evaluation will illuminate an author's reasons for taking a particular stance on an issue and will aid in readers' evaluation of the author's ideas.

It is our hope that these books will give readers a deeper understanding of the issues debated and an appreciation of the complexity of even seemingly simple issues when good and honest people disagree. This awareness is particularly important in a democratic society such as ours in which people enter into public debate to determine the common good. Those with whom one disagrees should not be regarded as enemies but rather as people whose views deserve careful examination and may shed light on one's own.

Thomas Jefferson once said that "difference of opinion leads to inquiry, and inquiry to truth." Jefferson, a broadly educated man, argued that "if a nation expects to be ignorant and free . . . it expects what never was and never will be." As individuals and as a nation, it is imperative that we consider the opinions of others and examine them with skill and discernment. The Opposing Viewpoints series is intended to help readers achieve this goal.

David L. Bender and Bruno Leone,
Founders

Introduction

"What is driving the demand for alternative medicine? Clearly science is not the driving force. Hospitals put alternative medicine clinics on their campuses because marketing surveys reveal intense public interest in the field, not because proven science demands them. Alternative therapies like Ayurvedic medicine, healing touch, and energy medicine may challenge the biomechanical theory of disease that has governed medical science for over a century, but they do not come close to overthrowing it.

Ronald W. Dworkin,
Policy Review, August–September 2001.

The modern fascination with herbal supplements, massage therapy, naturopathy, and other forms of complementary and alternative medicine (CAM) is not a unique phenomenon in U.S. history. The country has witnessed at least two other waves of interest in unconventional healing. The first took place in the decades leading up to the Civil War when temperance leagues and religious reformers wanted to cleanse Americans of bad habits, including poor health. A bit skeptical of the power of institutional medicine and open to the ways of frontier doctors who often relied on natural remedies, several reformers touted alternative ways of addressing illness. Some advocated homeopathy, which claimed that illnesses could be cured by giving patients miniscule amounts of substances known to cause similar symptoms in well people. Others supported hydropathy, a school of thought that included the use of cold water immersion as well as the adoption of proper eating and dressing habits to fend off disease. Still others took to prescribing herbs, which were as likely to cure ailments as many of the patented and unpatented medicines that were sold around the country. Learning herbal cures from Native American tribes, Constantine Samuel Rafinesque (1783–1840) founded "eclectic medicine," a hybrid that incorporated traditional remedies as well as newer medical practices in the hope that the number of options would provide doctors with at least one viable cure for whatever complaints patients had.

The second period of interest in alternative medicine arrived at the end of the nineteenth century. The popularity of chiropractic treatments, naturopathy, and other alternative healthcare therapies at this time was primarily a result of people's dissatisfaction with the risks of conventional treatments. For example, the relatively new practice of vaccination faced opposition because of the number of deaths attributed to improperly stored and administered doses. In addition, mid-nineteenth-century reformers such as physician Russell Thacher Trall (1812–1877) noted that conventional drugs oftentimes made patients sicker rather than curing them of their illnesses. Trall believed that improved diet, hydropathy, and even changing the mindset of patients would do more to relieve ailments than to focus on treating symptoms with drugs. His views helped shape the "drugless healing" movement that surfaced in the late nineteenth century. Advocates of this movement were dismayed at conventional doctors' inattention to the emotional state of their patients and consequently campaigned for a holistic medical approach that would treat the whole person rather than just his or her physical symptoms.

The reemergence of alternative medicine in modern times has its roots in these past waves of interest. Although conventional medicine has become more sophisticated, highly regulated, and quite effective, those who turn to CAM therapies today still harbor a distrust of institutionalized care. Some of this distrust can be attributed to the experimentation of the

1960s, when all forms of authority fell under scrutiny, and many wanted a return to nature and ancient traditions in the face of increasingly depersonalized modernization. But part of the explanation for CAM's popularity can also be traced to much earlier complaints about the lack of personalized care and the intention of people to take charge of their own well-being by focusing on preventative measures that do not involve an embrace of manufactured drugs.

One reason people are looking into preventative medicine is the rising costs of health care. Because many Americans are unable to afford insurance or struggle with poor coverage, herbal supplements, massage, and other forms of alternative medicine present themselves as a relatively inexpensive means of warding off serious illness as well as the high costs of doctor visits and hospital stays. In a 2006 interview conducted for the Internet press release site *PR9.net*, alternative medicine advocate Brenda Skidmore states, "For the working class poor CAM is gaining popularity and viewed as a 'last hope' for chronic illness. Besides CAM is becoming more widely accepted by conventional medicine and is often being used alongside with what has been considered standard treatments."

The "complementary" aspect of CAM has indeed become important to those who wish to see its greater acceptance in American society. Chiropractors, naturopaths, and other CAM practitioners believe that instead of setting themselves apart from conventional medicine, they wish to see greater integration between the two schools with the objective of offering the best of both disciplines to their patients. In some respects, this move toward integrative medicine may be an attempt to find legitimacy through acceptance. CAM supporters, however, argue that there is a place for both forms of care—or that the dichotomy is itself misleading because any method of healing a patient is a valid practice in the broad field of medicine. Most advocates of alternative medicine, for example, attest that acute pain and trauma are best remedied by surgery or conventional drugs, while those that suffer chronic ailments are better served by natural, preventative techniques and medicines. In a 2003 issue of the *Journal of Alternative and Complementary Medicine*, Bruce Barrett points out that patients are happy to avail themselves of whatever works. He cites several studies that show that "many patients want access to both conventional and CAM therapies." He also adds "that a significant number of their conventional clinicians appear supportive."

Many conventional healthcare practitioners have shown interest in CAM treatments for various reasons. Some have been intrigued by the clinically unexplored potential of remedies that have remained a vital part of world medicine for centuries. Others have come to accept the fact that they need to be familiar with the types of treatments their patients are experimenting with and sometimes preferring. In a 2005 issue of *Applied Neurology*, neurologist Alexander Mauskop, director of the New York Headache Clinic, was paraphrased as saying that doctors "'have no choice' but to become informed about integrative medicine for the simple reason that not being in the loop can have an adverse impact on their practices."

Staying abreast of patients' alternative therapies out of curiosity or for business reasons, however, is quite different from endorsing or even prescribing CAM treatments. Conventional healthcare workers' beliefs in the effectiveness of alternative medicine are quite diverse, and thus there is a great deal of controversy in the profession over the ethics of tolerating CAM or silently approving of it by refusing to label it as pseudoscience. Some doctors recognize that patients tend to seek alternative treatments for chronic illnesses—such as arthritis, recurring pain, and allergies—for which medical science has no cure. In a well-known 1998 article for *The Scientist*, Walter A. Brown, a clinical professor of psychiatry, acknowledges that alternative medicines and therapies have a value in such cases because they can do what science cannot—they can make patients feel better. "The catch is, like most treatments of the past and many conventional treatments of today, most alternative therapies probably have no intrinsic therapeutic value; their benefit comes from the placebo effect; more precisely, the healing situation," Brown contends. "Although people with these afflictions may or may not benefit from the manipulation of energy fields, herbal concoctions, huge doses of vitamins, or alterations in the flow of chi they so fervently embrace, they almost certainly benefit from the reassurance, hope, and relief of distress that comes from being in a healing situation."

Opponents of this tolerant view argue that deceiving patients with treatments that have no therapeutic value other than to relieve distress is not the role of physicians. To them, doctors need to treat the sick with evidence-based therapies that could have a chance of succeeding in thwarting an illness. Other critics maintain that giving validity to CAM treatments in the medical field only diverts research funding from more likely cures. Thus, the more money spent studying inconclusive treatments such as acupuncture and homeopathy, the less money spent finding potent AIDS drugs or verifiable cancer treatments.

Despite such resistance, CAM classes are part of the curriculum of many medical schools across the country. The federal government has also established the National Center for Complementary and Alternative Medicine (NCCAM) to study the potential medicinal uses of everything from crystal therapies to herbal supplements. This institutionalization of alternative medicine further attests to its popularity and, in turn, validates its use so that it gains even more adherents. The most recent government statistics as of 2007 indicate that roughly 36 percent of Americans who are 18 years and older use some form of alternative medicine. The National Center for Health Statistics director, Edward J. Sondik, says that these numbers reinforce the notion that Americans are becoming somewhat dissatisfied with aspects of conventional medicine—whether for cost, lack of sympathy, or some other complaint. He concludes, "What we see is that a sizable percentage of the public puts their personal health into their own hands."

In *Opposing Viewpoints: Alternative Medicine,* several authors discuss the growing popularity of alternative medicine in the United States. Some view it as a positive trend that illustrates both the power of personal choice and the healthy broadening of medicine to include holistic treatments that have been around for a long time. Others view CAM's expansion with trepidation, noting that popular belief in nonscientific medical practices undermines rational thinking and sets dangerous precedents for deceptive and potentially harmful quackery. These and other controversies surrounding the growth of alternative medicine are examined in *Opposing Viewpoints: Alternative Medicine.* The collected viewpoints address the rise of alternative medicine in this most recent period of popular interest and explore the consequences of CAM's growing acceptance.

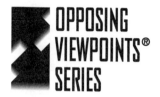
**OPPOSING
VIEWPOINTS®
SERIES**

CHAPTER 1

Does Alternative Medicine Work?

Chapter Preface

M any medical practitioners who use complementary and alternative medicine (CAM) believe that it is useful in treating chronic pain, stress, and other health problems. These professionals are convinced that CAM could be very helpful in the medical field, especially in the area of preventative health care, if it were more widely accepted by the medical community. They also are quick to note the limitations of alternative treatements and emphasize its "complementary" nature. For example, neurologist Shri Mishra of the Keck School of Medicine at the University of Southern California maintains: "If you're having a stroke, I'm not going to give you yoga therapy, but many of the complementary and alternative modalities have a great deal to offer in health promotion and disease prevention, and the very important role they play is to complement. For many illnesses that feature rehabilitative problems, there is a real need for complementary and alternative modalities, which really are usually about lifestyle, healthy living."

Mishra is one of several physicians who are hoping to bring greater acceptance of CAM by judging its merits in standardized tests and controlled trials. In an interview with *Applied Neurology*, neurologist Allan C. Bowling asserted: "There is a lot of interest and excitement in how these therapies can be applied, but we still need the hard evidence to really have them be completely integrated. We have to see evidence that they actually work." Achieving validity is time consuming, however, as clinical trials are usually conducted over years. In addition, some proponents of alternative medicine claim that research for this field is under-funded because of institutional prejudice against it. Despite research handicaps, some trials have moved forward, and a few have shown that alternative therapies have worked better than placebos (purposefully ineffective treatments or medicines given to experimental control groups).

Such findings, however, do not convince everyone that CAM has a medical value. In 2005, the *Lancet*, a prestigious British medical journal, referred to homeopathy, for instance, as "nothing but a placebo." Many other alternative practices and remedies such as herbal medicines, acupuncture, and chiropractic treatments have also been derided by conventional physicians. Most critics assert that the only healthful properties of CAM are not in the medicines and therapies themselves but in the minds of those patients who want to believe in their efficacy. They insist that, without clinical proof, the medical profession cannot afford to delude patients by prescribing treatments that have no ability to heal the physical symptoms of patients' ailments.

In the following chapter, both proponents and detractors of various CAM practices debate the value of these treatments.

| "Homeopaths have found and verified that whatever a substance has been found to cause, it will also cure in specially prepared homeopathic doses."

Homeopathic Medicine Is Effective

Dana Ullman

In the following viewpoint, Dana Ullman, MPH (Master of Public Health), describes how homeopaths use the "principle of similars" to treat ailments by giving patients incredibly small doses (nano-doses) of a substance known to cause that ailment in a well person. Ullman explains that this practice has been used outside the conventional medical field for two hundred years and has, in the past few decades, been proven effective in structured trials. Ullman, the author of several books on homeopathic medicine, operates an online homeopathic question-and-answer and retail Web site at www.homeopathic.com.

As you read, consider the following questions:

1. According to Ullman, why do homeopaths reject the notion that alleviating symptoms of illness is beneficial to healing?

2. What are "drug provings," as Ullman defines them?

3. As Ullman explains, how is the concept of "resonance" involved in homeopathic treatment?

The word "homeopathy" is derived from two Greek words: *homoios* which means "similar" and *pathos* which means "suffering." Homeopathy's basic premise is called the "principle of similars," and it refers to recurrent observation and experience that a medicinal substance will elicit a healing response for the specific syndrome of symptoms (or suffering) that it has been proven to cause when given to a healthy person in overdose.

The beauty of the principle of similars is that it not only initiates a healing response, but it encourages a respect for the body's wisdom. Because symptoms represent the best efforts of our body in its defenses against infection or stress, it makes sense to utilize a medicine that helps and mimics this defense rather than that inhibits or suppresses it. The principle of similars may be one of nature's laws that, when used well, can be one of our most sophisticated healing strategies. . . .

The Underlying Basis of Modern Physiology and Homeopathy

The underlying principle of homeopathy is also at the heart of modern physiology. It is commonly understood in medicine today [as of 2005] that symptoms are not just something "wrong" with the body, but rather, they represent the efforts of the body and mind to defend and heal itself from a variety of infective agents and/or stresses. The body creates fever, inflammation, pain, discharge, or whatever is necessary in order to heal itself. While these symptoms represent the body's best efforts to heal, they are not always successful in doing so. Ultimately, homeopathic medicines are some of the most powerful natural drugs available today to help augment the body's ability to heal itself.

Medical science today is increasingly recognizing symptoms as adaptive responses of the body. Standard texts of pathology define the process of inflammation as the manner in which the body seeks to wall off, heat up, and burn out infective agents or foreign matter. The cough has long been known as a protective mechanism for clearing breathing passages. Diarrhea has been shown to be a defensive effort of the body to remove pathogens or irritants more quickly from the colon. Discharges are understood as the body's way of ridding itself of dead bacteria, viruses, and cells. Even high blood pressure is an important defense and adaptation to the internal and external stresses that a person experiences.

The derivation of the word "symptom" is helpful to better understanding of the disease process and the healing process. The word "symptom" comes from a Greek root and refers to "something that falls together with something else." Symptoms are a "sign" or a "signal" of something else, and treating them doesn't necessarily change that "something else." Just because a drug gets rid of a symptom does not mean that the person is cured. In fact, drugs that suppress or inhibit a symptom tend to provide only a guise of success and usually lead to a longer and more serious illness. Using drugs to suppress symptoms is akin to pulling the plug on your car's oil pressure warning light. Just because the light is turned off doesn't mean that your car's oil pressure is "cured." In fact, ignoring that light may lead to your car's breakdown. . . .

Once one recognizes that symptoms are important and useful defenses of the body, it makes less sense to use drugs that inhibit or suppress this wisdom of the body. Instead of using drugs to suppress symptoms, it makes sense to use medicines to strengthen the body's own defense system so that the body can more effectively heal itself. Here is where it makes sense to use homeopathic medicines.

Medicines That Respect the Wisdom of the Body

The use of the principle of similars in healing actually has ancient roots. In the 4th century B.C., Hippocrates is known to have said, "Through the like, disease is produced, and through the application of the like it is cured." The famed Delphic Oracle in Greece proclaimed the value of the law of similars, stating, "that which makes sick shall heal." Paracelsus, a well-known 16th century physician and alchemist, used the law of similars extensively in practice and referred to it in writings. His formulation of the "Doctrine of Signatures" spoke directly of the value in using similars in healing. He affirmed, "You there bring together the same anatomy of the herbs and the same anatomy of the illness into one order. This simile gives you understanding of the way in which you shall heal."

This principle of similars (using a substance to treat the similar symptoms that it causes) is also used in conventional medicine, with immunizations being the most obvious example, that is, small doses of a "weakened" pathogen are used to prevent what larger doses cause. None other than the "father of immunology," Dr. Emil Adolph Von Behring (1906), directly pointed to the origins of immunizations when he asserted, "By what technical term could we more appropriately speak of this influence than by Hahnemann's word 'homeopathy.'" (Samuel Hahnemann, MD, 1755–1843, was a renowned German physician and the founder of homeopathy.) Modern allergy treatment, likewise, utilizes the homeopathic approach by the use of small doses of allergens in order to create an antibody response.

Conventional medical treatment also uses homeopathy's principle of similars in choosing radiation to treat people with cancer (radiation causes cancer), digitalis for heart conditions (digitalis creates heart conditions), and Ritalin for hyperactive children (Ritalin is an amphetamine-like drug which normally causes hyperactivity). Other examples are the use of nitroglycerine for heart conditions, gold salts for arthritic conditions, and colchicine for gout, all of which are known to cause the similar symptoms that they are found to treat. . . .

It should be acknowledged that although the conventional medical treatments mentioned above may be homeopathic-like, they do not follow other fundamental principles of homeopathy. Immunizations and allergy treatments are given to prevent or cure special ailments, while homeopathic medicines are substances individually prescribed based on the overall syndrome of body and mind symptoms the person is experiencing, and therefore a homeopathic medicine is thought to strengthen the person's overall body-mind constitution, not just to prevent or treat a specific illness. Also, these conventional medical treatments are not individually prescribed to the high degree of selectivity that is common in homeopathy, and they are not prescribed in as small or as safe a dose.

And speaking of dose, this subject is vital, and homeopaths have uncovered an amazing and initially confusing power of the human organism. Homeopaths have found that sick people develop hypersensitivity to substances that cause the similar symptoms that they are experiencing. Further, by giving very small doses of this substance, a person can and will experience an immunological and therapeutic benefit without a toxic burden.

Determining What a Medicine Can Cure

For over 200 years, hundreds of thousands of homeopaths throughout the world have carefully catalogued and now computerized the idiosyncratic physical, emotional, and mental symptoms that thousands of substances have caused in healthy people. . . . Homeopaths have thereby created the most extensive body of toxicological information available today, though this information focuses on the symptoms that these substance cause, not on the dose in which they cause them. Homeopaths have found and verified that whatever a substance has been found to cause, it will also cure in specially prepared homeopathic doses.

Thousands of substances have undergone toxicological studies, which homeopaths call "drug provings." These experiments are conducted on human subjects, not animals, to determine what various substances from the plant, mineral, animal, or chemical kingdom cause in overdose. Homeopaths have found that these experiments lay the foundation for what symptoms each substance causes and, thus, what affinity each substance has to the human body.

Then, when homeopaths see patients, they obtain the unique and detailed symptomatological history of each patient and seek to find the specific substance from the plant, mineral, animal, or chemical kingdom that would cause the similar syndrome of symptoms that the patient is experiencing. It is not surprising that large numbers of homeopaths throughout the world today use sophisticated expert system software to help them individualize medicinal substances to their patients.

After finding a match between a substance's toxicology and the patient's specific symptom pattern, the homeopath gives a specially prepared microdose of this medicinal agent. . . .

Nano-doses, Powerful Results

Homeopathic medicine presents a significantly different pharmacological approach to treating sick people. Instead of using strong and powerful doses of medicinal agents that have a broad-spectrum effect on a wide variety of people with a similar disease, homeopaths use extremely small doses of medicinal substances that are highly individualized to a person's physical and psychological syndrome of disease, not simply an assumed localized pathology.

Homeopathic medicines are so small in dose that it is appropriate to refer to them as a part of the newly defined field of "nanopharmacology" (the prefix "nano" derives from Latin and means dwarf; today, the prefix is used to refer to "nano-technology" or the "nanosciences" which explores the use of extremely small technologies or processes, at least one-billionth of a unit, designated as 10^{-9}). To understand the nature and the degree of homeopathy's nanopharmacology, it is important to know the following characteristics of how homeopathic medicines are made.

Making Homeopathic Medicines

1. Most homeopathic medicines are made by diluting a medicinal substance in a double-distilled water. It should be noted that physicists who study the properties of water commonly acknowledge that water has many mysterious and amazing properties. Because homeopaths use a double-distilled water, it is highly purified, enabling the medicinal substance to solely infiltrate and imprint the water. . . .

2. Each substance is diluted, most commonly, 1 part of the original medicinal agent to 9 or 99 parts double-distilled water. The mixture is then vigorously stirred or shaken. The solution is then diluted again 1:9 or 1:99 and vigorously shaken. This process of consecutive diluting and shaking or stirring is repeated 3, 6, 12, 30, 200, 1,000, or even 1,000,000 times. Simply "diluting" the medicines without vigorously shaking them doesn't activate the medicinal effects.

3. It is inaccurate to say that homeopathic medicines are extremely diluted; they are extremely "potentized." "Potentization" refers to the specific process of sequential dilution with vigorous shaking. Each consecutive dilution infiltrates the new double-distilled water and imprints upon it the fractal form of the original substance used (fractal refers to the specific consecutively smaller pattern or form within a larger pattern). Ultimately,

some type of fractal or hologram of the original substance may be imprinted in the water.

4. Scientists at several universities and hospitals in France and Belgium have discovered that the vigorous shaking of the water in glass bottles causes extremely small amounts of silica fragments or "chips" to fall into the water. In fact, these researchers found that high amounts (6 parts per million) of released silica infiltrate the water. These "silica chips" may help to store the information in the water, with each medicine that is initially placed in the water creating its own pharmacological effect.

Over 200 years of experience by homeopaths throughout the world has shown that the more that a substance undergoes potentization (the process of sequential dilution with vigorous shaking in-between each dilution), the more powerful the medicine becomes, the longer it acts, and the less doses are generally needed. Because of these observations and experiences, homeopaths refer to medicines that have been potentized 200 times or more as "high potencies" and those that have been potentized less than 12 times as "low potencies."

In this light, homeopaths insist that their medicines are NOT extremely small doses. Instead, they assume that the double-distilled and purified water is changed and becomes imprinted and activated.

Homeopaths will be the first to acknowledge that their medicine will not have any effect at all, unless the person taking them has a hypersensitivity to the medicine. A person will have this hypersensitivity if and when they exhibit the syndrome of symptoms that the substance has previously been found to cause.

Still, it is admittedly difficult to initially accept the possibility that such nanopharmacological doses can have any effect at all. And yet, some highly respected basic scientific research has begun to verify the claims that homeopaths have made since its inception in the 1800s.

Principle and Power of Resonance

Before discussing these scientific studies, it may be helpful to make brief reference to a subject for which there is common knowledge. Basic principles of physics teach us that hypersensitivity exists when there is "resonance." An example from music is helpful here: Whenever a "C" note is played on a piano (or any instrument), other "C" notes reverberate, while other notes are not affected at all. Even when one instrument is relatively far away from another, its C strings will reverberate when a C note is played.

Ultimately, homeopathy is a medical system based on resonance (commonly referred to as the "principle of similars"). Two hundred years of experience by hundreds of thousands of homeopaths have consistently discovered that specially prepared, extremely small doses of medicine can powerfully augment a person's healing response when there is a similarity between the toxicology of the medicine and the symptom complex of the sick person. One of the special features of homeopathy is that whenever a patient is given a homeopathic medicine that does not match his or her symptoms, nothing happens. But when there is a match, people experience significant improvement in their overall health. . . .

A History of Efficacy

Homeopathy first developed a significant popularity in Europe and the United States primarily because of the astounding successes it experienced in treating people suffering from the various infectious disease epidemics in the 19th century. The death rates in the homeopathic hospitals from cholera, scarlet fever, typhoid, yellow fever, pneumonia, and others was typically one-half to even one-eighth of conventional medical hospitals. Similar good results were also observed in mental institutions and prisons under the care of homeopathic physicians compared to those under the care of conventional doctors. These consistent and significant results could not be attributed to a placebo effect. In other words, there is clear empirical evidence that homeopathic medicines were highly effective in treating various infectious diseases and in psychiatric disorders.

Unfortunately, conventional physicians and scientists have continually provided misinformation about the status of scientific evidence about homeopathic medicine. They have frequently and incorrectly asserted that there is no research to prove that homeopathic medicines work, and they further have asserted that there is no way that the extremely small doses can have any effect whatsoever.

This type of statement simply reflects ignorance of the scientific literature. It is remarkable to note that some of the earliest placebo-controlled and double-blinded studies ever performed were actually conducted by homeopathic physicians. . . .

Controlled Studies

An independent group of physicians and scientists evaluated homeopathic clinical research prior to October 1995. They reviewed 186 studies, 89 of which met their pre-defined criteria for their meta-analysis. They found that on average patients given a homeopathic medicine were 2.45 times more likely to have experienced a clinically beneficial effect. When reviewing only the highest quality studies and when adjusting for publication bias, the researchers found that subjects given a homeopathic medicine were still 1.86 times more likely to experience improved health as compared with those given a placebo. The researchers have also noted that it is extremely common in conventional medical research for more rigorous trials to yield less positive results than less rigorous trials.

Homepoathic Medicine vs. Conventional Medicine	
Homeopathic Medicine	**Conventional Medicine**
Illness	
Is an individual expression of imbalance and has important meaning	Occures in well-defined groups based on pathology, and meaning of illness is irrelevant
Symptoms	
Are evidence of disharmony and the person's attempt to restore order	Are bad
Are analyzed to follow progress of treatment	Successful treatment makes them go away
Diagnosis	
The understanding of the phenomenon of the illness	The search for the structural cause
The whole person is taken into account	
Treatment	
Individualized and based on the entire expression of symptoms	Based on the pathologic diagnosis
Self-care (what the client does) is emphasized	What the doctor does is emphasized
Based on like cures and potentized microdoses of medicines	Based on opposing and suppressing symptoms, and high doses of medicine

TAKEN FROM: "Principles of Homeopathy."
www.holisticonline.com/Homeopathy.

The most important question that good scientists pose about any clinical research is: have there been replications of clinical studies by independent researchers? When at least three independent researchers verify the efficacy of a treatment, it is considered to be a valid and effective treatment.

Four separate bodies of researchers have conducted clinical trials in the use of a homeopathic medicine (Oscillococcinum 200C) in the treatment of influenza-like syndromes. Each of these trials was relatively large in the number of subjects (487, 300, 100, and 372), and all were multi-centered placebo-controlled and double-blinded (two of the three trials were also randomized). Each of these trials showed statistically significant results.

One other body of research in the use of Galphimia glauca in the treatment of hay fever was replicated successfully seven times, but this research was conducted by the same group of researchers, and thus far, this work has not been conducted by any other researchers.

A body of clinical research in homeopathy that has been consistently recognized as some of the highest quality scientific research has been conducted by a group of researchers at the University of Glasgow and Glasgow Homeopathic Hospital. They conducted four studies on people suffering from various respiratory allergies (hay fever, asthma, and perennial allergic rhinitis). In total, they treated 253 patients and found a 28% improvement in visual analogue scores in those given a homeopathic medicine, as compared with a 3% improvement in patients given a placebo (P=.0007)(The "P" refers to the "probability" of these results occurring simply by chance, and thus, the lower the number, the greater the likelihood that the treatment used is effective. When "P" equals .05, this means that there are 5 chances out of 100 that the effective of a specific treatment happened by chance, and scientists today consider this 5% chance as adequate evidence of a treatment's effectiveness. In this study, however, there was an extremely high likelihood that the treatment was effective because there were only seven chances out of 10,000 (!) that this result happened by chance.) . . .

One other study is worth mentioning. This study was on 53 patients with fibromyalgia, which is a newly recognized syndrome that includes musculoskeletal symptoms, fatigue, and insomnia. Participants given individually chosen homeopathic treatment showed significantly greater improvements in tender point count and tender point pain, quality of life, global health and a trend toward less depression compared with those on placebo. "Helpfulness from treatment" in homeopathic patients as compared to those given a placebo was very significant (P=.004). What is also extremely interesting about this study was that the researchers found that people on homeopathic treatment also experienced changes in EEG [electro-encephalogram] readings. Not only did subjects who were given a homeopathic medicine experience improved health, they were shown to experience different changes in the brain wave activity. This evidence of clinical benefits and objective physiological action from homeopathic medicines in people with chronic symptoms constitutes very strong evidence that these nanodoses can have observable effects.

One of the most significant studies showing the power of homeopathic medicines was in the treatment of people with chronic obstructive pulmonary disease (COPD). COPD is a general term for a group of respiratory ailments and is the fourth leading cause of death in the U.S. Chronic bronchitis and emphysema are two conditions that are included in the more broad diagnosis of COPD.

A prospective, randomized, double-blind, placebo-controlled study with parallel assignment was performed to assess the influence of sublingually administered Kali bichromicum (potassium dichromate) 30C on the amount of tenacious, stringy tracheal secretions in critically ill patients with a history of tobacco use and COPD. In this study, 50 patients received either Kali bichromicum 30C globules (group 1) or placebo (group 2). This study found a very substantial improvement in the health of patients given this homeopathic medicine. Further, the time that these patients needed to be in the hospital was reduced by almost 50%, and their need for additional treatment to help with their breathing was dramatically reduced. . . .

Possible Explanations for Nano-Doses

Precisely how homeopathic medicines work remains a mystery according to present scientific thinking. And yet, despite the paradox of homeopathic medicines, nature and new technologies are replete with striking examples of the powerful effects from extremely small doses.

It is commonly known that certain species of moths can smell pheromones of its own species up to two miles in distance. It is no simple coincidence that species only sense pheromones from those in the same species who emit them (akin to the homeopathic principle of similars), as though they have developed exquisite and specific receptor sites for what they need to survive and to propagate their species. Likewise, sharks are known to sense blood in the water at distances, and when one considers the volume of water in the ocean, it becomes obvious that sharks, like all living creatures, develop extreme hypersensitivity for whatever will help ensure their survival.

It is therefore not surprising that renowned astronomer Johann Kepler once said, "Nature uses as little as possible of anything."

One metaphor that may help us understand how and why extremely small doses of medicinal agents may work derives from present knowledge of modern submarine radio communications. Normal radio waves simply do not penetrate water, so submarines must use an extremely low frequency radio wave. However, the terms "extremely low" are inadequate to describe this specific situation because radio waves used by submarines to penetrate water are so low that a single wavelength is typically several miles long!

If one considers that the human body is 70–80% water, perhaps the best way to provide pharmacological information to the body and into intercellular fluids is with nanodoses. Like the above mentioned extremely low frequency radio waves, it may be necessary to use extremely low (and activated) doses as used in homeopathic medicines, in order for a person to receive the medicinal effect.

It is important to understand that nanopharmacological doses will not have any effect unless the person is hypersensitive to the specific medicinal substance. Hypersensitivity is created when there is some type of resonance between the medicine and the person. Because the system of homeopathy bases its selection of the medicine on its ability to cause in overdose the similar symptoms that the sick person is experiencing, homeopathy's "principle of similars" is simply a practical method of finding the substance to which a person is hypersensitive.

The homeopathic principle of similars makes further sense when one considers that modern physiologists and pathologists recognize that disease is not simply the result of breakdown or surrender of the body but that symptoms are instead representative of the body's efforts to fight infection or adapt to stress.

Using a nanodose that is able to penetrate deeply into the body and that is specifically chosen for its ability to mimic the symptoms that the sick person is experiencing helps to initiate a profound healing process. It is also important to highlight the fact that a homeopathic medicine is not simply chosen for its ability to cause a similar disease that a person has but for its ability to cause a similar syndrome of symptoms of disease, of which the specific localized disease is a part. By understanding that the human body is a complex organism that creates a wide variety of physical and psychological symptoms, homeopaths acknowledge biological complexity and have a system of treatment to deal with it.

Although no one knows precisely how homeopathic medicines initiate the healing process, there is over 200 years of experience by hundreds of thousands of clinicians and tens of millions of patients that these medicines they have powerful effects. One cannot help but sense and anticipate the veritable treasure-trove of knowledge that further research in homeopathy and nanopharmacology will bring in this new millennium.

> "Homeopaths have had over 200 years to demonstrate their wares and have failed to do so."

Homeopathic Medicine Is Ineffective

Robert Todd Carroll

Robert Todd Carroll is the author of the Skeptic's Dictionary, *a print and online encyclopedia that focuses on debunking hoaxes, conspiracy theories, and unscientific or deceptive practices. In one of the entries, Carroll argues that homeopathic medicinal remedies are unproven and may even be dangerous. He claims that tests of homeopathic cures are unscientific and their abnormally high professed success rates make them even more suspicious. Carroll asserts that the usefulness of homeopathic treatments may have more to do with their calming psychological effect than their physiological impact. But he warns that an unquestioning belief in their effectiveness may be dangerous because it may prevent seriously sick individuals from seeking appropriate medical care.*

As you read, consider the following questions:

1. What is Samuel Hahnemann's practice of "dynamization," according to Carroll?

Robert Todd Carroll, *skepdic.com*, Hoboken, NJ: John Wiley & Sons, 2007. Copyright © 2007 Robert Todd Carroll. Reprinted with permission of John Wiley & Sons, Inc.

2. Why was Samuel Hahnemann's empirical testing method flawed, in Carroll's opinion?

3. What is the "placebo effect," and how does Carroll tie it to the possible benefits of homeopathy?

Classical homeopathy originated in the 19th century with Samuel Christian Friedrich Hahnemann (1755–1843) as an alternative to the standard medical practices of the day, such as phlebotomy or bloodletting. Opening veins to bleed patients, force disease out of the body, and restore the humors to a proper balance was a popular medical practice until the late 19th century Hahnemann rejected the notion that disease should be treated by letting out the offensive matter causing the illness. Instead, he argued that disease should be treated by helping the vital force restore the body to harmony and balance. He rejected other common medical practices of his day such as purgatives and emetics "with opium and mercury-based calomel" [as medical historian Guy Williams writes]. In retrospect, Hahnemann's alternative medicine was more humane and less likely to cause harm than many of the conventional practices of his day. . . .

Setting Homeopathy Apart

Hahnemann put forth his ideas of disease and treatment in *The Organon of Homeopathic Medicine* (1810) and *Theory of Chronic Diseases* (1821). The term 'homeopathy' is derived from two Greek words: *homeo* (similar) and *pathos* (suffering). Hahnemann meant to contrast his method with the convention of his day of trying to balance "humors" by treating a disorder with its opposite (*allos*). He referred to conventional practice as allopathy. Even though modern scientific medicine bears no resemblance to the theory of balancing humors or treating disease with its opposite, modern homeopaths and other advocates of "alternative" medicine misleadingly refer to today's conventional physicians as allopaths.

Classical homeopathy is generally defined as a system of medical treatment based on the use of minute quantities of remedies that in larger doses produce effects similar to those of the disease being treated. Hahnemann believed that very small doses of a medication could have very powerful healing effects because their potency could be affected by vigorous and methodical shaking (succussion). Hahnemann referred, to this alleged increase in potency by vigorous shaking as *dynamization*. . . . Dynamization was for Hahnemann a process of releasing an energy that he regarded as essentially immaterial and spiritual. . . .

Healing through Harmonizing

Like most of his contemporaries, Hahnemann believed that health was a matter of balance and harmony, but for him it was the vital force, the spirit in the body, that did the balancing and harmonizing, that is, the healing.

Hahnemann claimed that most chronic diseases were caused by miasms and the worst of these miasms were the 'psora.' The evidence for the miasm theory, however, is completely absent and seems to have been the result of some sort of divine revelation. The word 'miasm' derives from the Greek and means something like "taint" or "contamination". Hahnemann supposed that chronic disease results from invasion of the body by one of the miasms through the skin. The first sign of disease is thus always a skin disorder of some kind.

His method of treatment might seem very modern: Find the right drug for the illness. However, his medicines were not designed to help the body fight off infection or rebuild tissue, but to help the vital spirit work its magic. . . .

Homeopathic Laws Are Not Empirically Testable

Homeopaths refer to "the Law of Infinitesimals" and the "Law of Similars" as grounds for using minute substances and for believing that like heals like, but these are not natural laws of science. If they are laws at all, they are metaphysical laws, i.e., beliefs about the nature of reality that would be impossible to test by empirical means. Hahnemann's ideas did originate in experience. That he drew metaphysical conclusions from empirical events does not, however, make his ideas empirically testable. The law of infinitesimals seems to have been partly derived from his notion that any remedy would cause the patient to get worse before getting better and that one could minimize this negative effect by significantly reducing the size of the dose. Most critics of homeopathy balk at this "law" because it leads to remedies that have been so diluted as to have nary a single molecule of the substance one starts with.

Hahnemann came upon his Law of Similars (like cures like) in 1790 while translating William Cullen's *Materia Medica* into German. He began experimenting on himself with various substances, starting with cinchona.

Daily for several days, he wrote, he had been taking four drams of the drug. Each time he had repeated the dose, his feet and finger tips had become cold, and other symptoms had followed which were typical of malaria. Each time he had stopped taking the cinchona, he had returned rapidly to a state of good health.

Hahnemann experimented on himself with various drugs over several years and concluded that "a doctor should use only those remedies which would have the power to create, in a healthy body, symptoms similar to those that might be seen in the sick person being treated" [Williams relates]. Medicines should be given in single doses, he claimed, not in complex mixtures. His conclusions seem to have been based upon intuition or revelation. He did not experiment with patients by giving them drugs to discover which remedies worked with which illnesses or that only unmixed substances were effective. Indeed, he couldn't experiment on sick people because he assumed the remedy must produce an effect similar to the disease and he'd never be able to tell what remedies to use be-

Homeopathy Is Unreliable

Proponents trumpet the few "positive" studies as proof that "homeopathy works." Even if their results can be consistently reproduced (which seems unlikely), the most that the study of a single remedy for a single disease could prove is that the remedy is effective against that disease. It would not validate homeopathy's basic theories or prove that homeopathic treatment is useful for other diseases.

Placebo effects can be powerful, of course, but the potential benefit of relieving symptoms with placebos should be weighed against the harm that can result from relying upon—and wasting money on—ineffective products. Spontaneous remission is also a factor in homeopathy's popularity. I believe that most people who credit a homeopathic product for their recovery would have fared equally well without it.

Stephen Barrett, "Homeopathy: The Ultimate Fake,"
Quackwatch, *December 28, 2003. www.quackwatch.com.*

cause the symptoms of the disease would be difficult to distinguish from those of the remedy in a sick person. Instead, he assumed that whatever caused the symptoms in a healthy person would be a remedy for a disease with similar symptoms.

The Flaws of "Proving"

Hahnemann's called this method of finding what symptoms a drug caused in a healthy person "proving."

Working on the principle of similarities, Hahnemann created remedies for various disorders that had symptoms similar to those of the substances his provers [test subject] had taken. However, [as one modern medical reviewer notes] "methods of proving are highly personalised and of individual relevance to the homoeopath or experimenter." In other words, one hundred homeopaths preparing a remedy for one patient might well come up with one hundred different remedies.

Hahnemann may be praised for empirically testing his medicines, but his method of testing is obviously flawed. He wasn't actually testing the medicines for effectiveness on sick people but for their effects on healthy people. In any case, he had to rely upon the subjective evaluations of his provers, all of whom were his disciples or family members and all of whom were interrogated by the master himself. But even if his data weren't tainted by the possibility of his suggesting symptoms to his provers or their reporting symptoms to impress or gain the approval of the master, it is a belief in magic that connects this list of symptoms with the cure of a disease with similar symptoms. In logic, this kind of leap of reasoning is called a non sequitur: It does not follow from the fact that drug A produces symptoms similar to disease B that taking A will relieve the symptoms of B. However, homeopaths take *customer satisfaction* with A as evidence that A works.

There is some evidence that Hahnemann did not use healthy subjects to prove any of the remedies he recommended for most disorders: sulfur, cuttlefish ink, salt, and sand.

What appears to have happened is that Hahnemann based his new provings largely on symptoms supposed to have been produced in his chronic patients. By his own rules this procedure was inadmissible, and in fact it undoubtedly led him to attribute to the effect of the medicines a number of symptoms that were really due to the diseases the patients were suffering from.

While we might excuse Hahnemann for not doing properly controlled experiments, we shouldn't be so generous toward modern homeopaths for not understanding the nature of anecdotes and testimonial evidence. However, we can't accuse them of not doing any properly designed controlled experiments. But we can blame them for not understanding some fundamental principles of evaluating the results of controlled experiments that involve giving drugs or even inert substances to humans.

Today's homeopaths should know that because of the complexity of each individual human body, fifty different people may react in fifty different ways to the same substance. This makes doing clinical trials on potential medicines a procedure that should rarely claim dramatic results on the basis of one set of trials. Finding a statistically significant difference, positive or negative, between an experimental (drug therapy) group and a control group in one trial of a drug should usually be taken with a grain of salt. So should *not* finding anything statistically significant. It is not uncommon for twenty trials of a drug to result in several with positive, several with negative, and several with mixed or inconclusive results.

Yet, despite the fact that of the hundreds of studies that have been done on homeopathic remedies the vast majority have found no value in the remedies, some defenders of homeopathy insist not only that homeopathic remedies work but they claim they know *how* they work. It seems, however, that scientists like Jacques Benveniste, who claim to know how homeopathy works, have put the cart before the horse. Benveniste claims to have proven that homeopathic remedies work by altering the structure of water, thereby allowing the water to retain a "memory" of the structure of the homeopathic substance that has been diluted out of existence (*Nature*, June 30, 1988). . . . Since homeopathic remedies don't work, there is no need for a theory as to *how* they work. What there is need of is an explanation for why so many people are satisfied with their homeopath despite all the evidence that homeopathic remedies are ineffective.

Why Some People Believe Homeopathy Works

Before attempting to explain why so many people believe homeopathy works, let me first defend the claim that homeopathic remedies are ineffective. There have been several reviews of various studies of the effectiveness of homeopathic treatments and not one of these reviews concludes that there is good evidence for *any* homeopathic remedy (HR) being effective. Homeopaths have had over 200 years to demonstrate their wares and have failed to do so. Sure, there are single studies that have found statistically significant differences between groups treated with an HR and control groups, but none of these have been replicated or they have been marred by methodological faults. Two hundred years and we're still waiting for proof! Having an open mind is one thing; waiting forever for evidence is more akin to wishful thinking. . . .

Nevertheless, homeopathy will always have its advocates, despite the lack of proof that its remedies are effective. Why? One reason is the prevalence of a misunderstanding of the causes of disease and how the human body deals with disease. Hahnemann was able to attract followers because he appeared to be a healer compared to those who were cutting veins or using poisonous purgatives to balance humors. More of his patients may have survived and recovered not because he healed them but because he didn't infect them or kill them by draining out needed blood or weaken them with strong poisons. Hahnemann's medicines were essentially nothing more than common liquids and were unlikely to cause harm in themselves. He didn't have to have too many patients survive and get better to look impressive compared to his competitors. If there is any positive effect on health it is not due to the homeopathic remedy, which is inert, but to the body's own natural curative mechanisms or to the belief of the patient (the placebo effect) or to the effect the manner of the homeopath has on the patient.

Stress can enhance and even cause illness. If a practitioner has a calming effect on the patient, that alone might result in a significant change in the feeling of well-being of the patient. And that feeling might well translate into beneficial physiological effects. The homeopathic method involves spending a lot of time with each patient to get a complete list of symptoms. It's possible this has a significant calming effect on some patients. This effect could enhance the body's own healing mechanisms in some cases. As homeopath Anthony Campbell puts it: "A homeopathic consultation affords the patient an opportunity to talk at length about her or his problems to an attentive and sympathetic listener in a structured environment, and this in itself is therapeutic." In other words, homeopathy is a form of psychotherapy. . . .

The Danger of Homeopathy

The main harm from classical homeopathy is not likely to come from its remedies, which are probably safe but ineffective, though this is changing as homeopathy becomes indiscernible from herbalism in some places. One potential danger is in the encouragement to self-diagnosis and treatment. Another danger lurks in not getting proper treatment by a conventional medical doctor in those cases where the patient could be helped by such treatment, such as for a bladder or yeast infection, or for cancer. Homeopathy might work in the sense of helping some people feel better some of the time. Homeopathy does not work, however, in the sense of explaining pathologies or their cures in a way which not only conforms with the data but which promises to lead us to a greater understanding of the nature of health and disease.

> "I personally believe chiropractic saves people from unnecessary surgeries and from taking too many pain medications."

Chiropractic Can Reduce Some Types of Pain

Michael Menke

In the following viewpoint, Dr. Michael Menke explains what he believes are the benefits of chiropractic medicine. He states that spinal manipulation can relieve some forms of back pain, neck pain, and other bodily aches. He is quick to note that chiropractic is not a cure-all, but he does believe that pain sufferers should consider such treatments before resorting to irreversible surgery. Menke is the first chiropractor appointed to the faculty of the Program in Integrative Medicine founded by Dr. Andrew Weil at the University of Arizona. He is also an author, teacher, and researcher.

As you read, consider the following questions:

1. What are the various ailments that chiropractic medicine might remedy, in Menke's experience and according to published reports?

2. When seeking treatment from a chiropractor, what does Menke suggest patients do instead of signing up for long term care?

3. Why does Menke believe that patients suffering from pain ought to seek a chiropractor first before electing to have corrective surgery?

D*rweil.com: What are the basic principles of chiropractic care?*

Michael Menke: Today, most people see chiropractors to reduce pain and to restore movement and improve function. But chiropractors have traditionally maintained a broader perspective on health than pain. Essentially, chiropractors encourage the body to heal itself by removing obstacles to healing. This is a hygienic principle: removing illness causes to improve health. Many chiropractors therefore offer nutritional and dietary advice, taking strain off muscles and joints, managing stress, and coaching patients in exercise, lifestyle and self-care.

Chiropractic was based upon the spine and its role in health and disease. This was not a novel idea when chiropractic was founded in 1895. In fact, the spine has held a role in health and disease in many cultures for thousands of years. Traditions granting the spine a role in health include: acupuncture and traditional Chinese medicine, Ayurvedic medicine, Eastern Hatha yoga and European bone-setters. In the late 19th century, both osteopathy (1874) and chiropractic (1895) emerged to carry on this tradition, each with a different emphasis.

Early chiropractors believed the spine could become "subluxated"—a minor slippage of vertebrae (backbone joints) that would pinch spinal nerves and cause all manner of diseases. The chiropractor's job was to remove subluxations by "adjusting" (manipulating) the spine to bring back normal movement, restore proper nerve flow and regain health.

The Body Can Heal Itself

When you go in for heart bypass surgery, the surgeon only fixes the valves of your pump, it is still up to your body to heal after surgery. The basis of chiropractic philosophy is much different from the surgical model. It is rooted in the simple notion that the body is able to heal itself. Chiropractic philosophy has always understood this simple fact: our bodies are so well designed that if you take care of them properly they will not only last you a lifetime, they will also function effortlessly and efficiently, without sacrificing strength, speed, or functioning well into the golden years. All they need is some good nutrition, water, and motion.

Mark Szostczuk,
"Philosophy of Chiropractic and Alternative Healing,"
New Life Journal, *July 2006.*

Though modern chiropractors still keep to the spine as their primary area of approach and many look for subluxations, most do not adhere to the concept that a subluxated spine is the only or the major cause of disease.

Practical Benefits

What kinds of ailments can chiropractors treat?

Chiropractic spinal manipulation has now had about three decades of very active research. Literally, hundreds of studies have been published in the major medical journals. Spinal manipulation has been found to be effective for some causes of low back pain (chronic pain more than acute), neck pain, muscle tension headaches, and a few other aches and pains.

From my own experience, chiropractic care can help some "slipped" (displaced) or degenerative disks of the spine. Carpal tunnel syndrome, if not too advanced, and other painful joints including knees, shoulders and elbows are sometimes helped with a chiropractic care or by co-management with another medical professional. There are also anecdotes of successful chiropractic treatment for middle ear infections, bedwetting and asthma through spinal adjusting. To date, these stories are not thoroughly researched. The persistence of these stories among chiropractic clinicians suggests that occasionally these conditions are helped, though each patient must be examined on a case-by-case basis. More research and clinical trials are needed to confirm just which of these cases are treatable by chiropractic management.

Dealing with a Reputable Chiropractor

How can people find a good chiropractor?

The best way to find a good chiropractor is to ask a friend or relative who goes to a reputable chiropractor. Another way is to ask your medical physician, dentist, optometrist, or other health care professional if he or she knows of any good chiropractors. Obviously the best referral is a satisfied patient who has been helped.

In a doctor of chiropractic, you look first for someone you can trust, as you would any of your health-care providers. I advise people to request an informational interview with a prospective chiropractor. You can then size up the office and the practitioner to see if everything seems plausible, comfortable and professional.

Never sign up for long-term programs, especially with upfront payments or payment plans. Make it clear that you are there to have your problem resolved, then you want to manage it yourself as soon as possible to prevent future problems. Ask for exercises and self-care instructions you can use at home or in the gym. (If your injury is bad or there is some arthritis, you may require more in-office treatment, maybe several times a year, to help you keep functioning.)

Finally, look for results. Chiropractic experts agree that if treated for more than two weeks without a change in your condition or you get worse, then your chiropractic treatment is not sufficient to your problem. You may discuss this with your chiropractor, seek the advice of another chiropractor, or try another health-care professional.

Sometimes it is difficult for you to judge your progress. This is especially true if you had pain for many years. At the beginning, your pain may seem slightly better, the same, or worse. But pain is not the primary indicator of improvement, especially at the beginning. Instead of focusing on pain, note how much more you can do. Improvement in activities of daily living is a more valid measure of progress than pain only. It is also reasonable to ask your medical physician for anti-inflammatory medication to help with discomfort while "rusty" joints regain movement and immobile ligaments are stretched. The chiropractor will also give you home-care instructions including icing, so in most cases you won't need medication.

A Non-Drug, Non-Surgical Approach

What do you say to people who are skeptical of chiropractic medicine?

Each health professional has expertise for helping some people with certain problems, but not everyone with every problem. I think we should all be skeptical informed consumers about health care. Chiropractic is a clinical service with its own limitations and risks like anything else. I personally believe chiropractic saves people from unnecessary surgeries and from taking too many pain medications. Old stories persist about chiropractors treating each and every disease by chiropractic adjustments, and the public knows that is nonsense. On the other hand, when people experience improvement with their headaches and low back pain, other benefits may also occur. With less pain and stress on the body, people can exercise more, work more, and be more sociable. Life is so much better without pain.

I think the bottom line is this: If you have pain that is not improving with your current self-care or treatment strategies, or you have a problem specifically related to your back, neck or spine, see if chiropractic can help. Don't wait until you have surgery to try chiropractic care. Once you have surgery, you are stuck with the results. Try chiropractic first because it offers non-drug, non-surgical approaches to some, but not all, health problems.

How did you become interested in being a chiropractor?

My father was spared a cervical fusion (neck vertebrae) surgery by his chiropractor, Joe Worz, in Greenville, Ohio, in the 1960s. My mother saw the chiropractor for occasional back pain. My first chiropractor in Dayton, Ohio, Harry Alexander, helped my severe neck pain after I fell off a tree at 30 years old, old enough to know better, you would think. At that time, I had degrees in psychology and behavioral sciences and was interested in how mind, body and spirit could work together to create better health. It was evident to me that strategies and models for how to be healthy were missing in most health care. Chiropractic aspired to a hygienic strategy, instead of treating disease. I also was intrigued with manual medicine to help reduce pain and improve people's lives. This perspective led me to my work with Dr. Weil's Program in Integrative Medicine here at the University of Arizona.

| "Chiropractic is a pseudoscientific approach to health care."

Chiropractic Is a Potentially Dangerous Pseudoscience

John Jackson

John Jackson is the director and administrator of UK-Skeptics, an Internet organization based in the United Kingdom that debunks pseudoscience, conspiracy theories, and paranormal phenomena. Jackson contends in the following viewpoint that chiropractic is a bogus medical practice that eschews scientific inquiry. In Jackson's opinion, chiropractic treatments are mainly ineffectual, but some pose real health threats. The risk of injury, coupled with the fact that chiropractors are now targeting children to increase their business clientele, makes chiropractic a dangerous alternative to conventional health care, Jackson maintains.

As you read, consider the following questions:

1. What is David Palmer's concept of "Innate Intelligence," according to Jackson?
2. How is "subluxation" a testable medical claim, as Jackson states?
3. As Jackson explains, what is the "dynamic thrust" treatment, and why is it dangerous?

Chiropractic was invented in 1895 by Canadian-born Daniel David Palmer, a medically unqualified layman. He had been a grocer before becoming a "magnetic healer" (transferring "healing energy" to patients by touching or waving hands over them) in Burlington, Iowa, USA.

He also dabbled in Phrenology (the belief in a relationship between the shape of a person's skull and their intelligence and personality), and he was influenced by mesmerism (a mystical healing force believed to work through hypnotic induction), spiritualism and vitalism. Vitalism is the belief in "vital energy" or a "spark of life" which distinguishes living from non-living matter; the same concept as its Chinese equivalent "chi" and its Indian equivalent "Prana".

Palmer called his vital energy: "Innate Intelligence". His belief was that this Innate Intelligence flowed through the body from the brain, through the spine, the nerves and on to the various organs of the body.

The theory of chiropractic which Palmer developed states that all disease is caused by the misalignment of vertebrae. A vertebra that is out of alignment, known as a "subluxation", blocks the natural flow of the vital "Innate Intelligence" through the body; thus leading to disease. . . .

Lack of Scientific Testing

Chiropractors claim to take a holistic approach to treatment, believing that the body is self-healing; although it sometimes needs help to heal itself. The human body does have a multitude of self-repair mechanisms, which have evolved naturally, and it does heal itself. Whether or not pseudoscientific intervention helps is open to question: a consideration that is applicable to all alternative treatments.

Most evidence that chiropractors put forward to back their claim is that of personal testimonies. This is not scientifically acceptable: even though someone may have felt they were

No Anatomical Evidence of Chiropractic Subluxation

There is plenty of room for the passage of spinal nerves and blood vessels through the fat-padded foraminal openings between the vertebrae. It cannot be imagined that slight displacement of a normal vertebra will place pressure on a spinal nerve. This was proven conclusively 25 years ago by experiments performed by Edmund S. Crelin, PhD, a prominent anatomist at Yale University. Using dissected spines with ligaments attached and the spinal nerves exposed, he used a drill press to bend and twist the spine. Using an ohm meter to record any contact between wired spinal nerves and the foraminal openings, he found that vertebrae could not be displaced enough to stretch or impinge a spinal nerve unless the force was great enough to break the spine. Crelin concluded [in a 1993 issue of *American Scientist*]: "This experimental study demonstrates conclusively that the subluxation of a vertebra as defined by chiropractic—the exertion of pressure on a spinal nerve which by interfering with the planned expression of Innate Intelligence produces pathology—does not occur."

Samuel Homola,
"How Chiropractic Subluxation Theory Threatens Public Health,"
Chirobase, *December 22, 2002. www.chirobase.org.*

helped by a chiropractic procedure, personal testimony is too unreliable to be considered as evidence.

In the 1997 *Journal of Canadian Chiropractic Association*, it was cited that 74% of chiropractors "do not accept the view that controlled clinical trials are the best way to validate chiropractic methods."

Controlled clinical trials are the method by which genuine treatments are differentiated from bogus ones. One of the hallmarks of a pseudoscience is that it fails to work under rigorous testing. The defence that scientific testing is not the way to test the claim is known as "special pleading"; it is another hallmark of pseudoscience.

The belief in "Innate Intelligence" often more simply referred to as "Innate" is a metaphysical belief and as such is not testable or scientific: it is a matter of faith.

Most pseudoscientific claims are untestable; however, the subluxation as a physical property lends itself to scientific testing. The fact of the matter is that chiropractors cannot even agree what a subluxation actually is, the original concept of misaligned vertebrae having lost favour with some in the field, perhaps because (x-ray) radiographs show no difference between before-treatment and after-treatment exposures.

There is no evidence that subluxations actually exist, never mind that they can be manipulated to cure disease or promote well-being. This is after more than a century of chiropractic's existence.

Misuse of Evidence

The one area that there is evidence that Chiropractic can be beneficial [according to a 1992 report by the RAND Corporation] is in treating lower-back pain ... although RAND are not so supportive of Chiropractic cervical (relating to the neck) spine manipulation.

Despite the fact that Chiropractors can achieve beneficial results using spinal manipulative therapy (SMT), this does not endorse Chiropractic itself: SMT is not unique to Chiropractic, it is also offered by qualified doctors and physiotherapists, for example. It is the inappropriate use of SMT that is the concern with Chiropractic.

The RAND report has been misused by chiropractors who have claimed that the RAND finding of SMT to be beneficial endorses Chiropractic itself. This is not the case. RAND spokesman, Dr. Paul Shekelle, released this statement in 1993:

... we have become aware of numerous instances where our results have been seriously misrepresented by chiropractors writing for their local paper or writing letters to the editor. ... RAND's studies were about spinal manipulation, not chiropractic, and dealt with appropriateness, which is a measure of net benefit and harms. Comparative efficacy of chiropractic and other treatments was not explicitly dealt with.

The Dangers of Chiropractic

• *The practitioners are not qualified doctors.*

Many people wrongly assume that chiropractors are a part of the medical community. They are not: they are a part of the alternative medicine industry. Unlike many other alternative practitioners, Chiropractors are thought by many to be medically qualified doctors, and as such people may place as much trust in their advice as they would in that of a qualified doctor.

• *Anti-vaccination stance.*

Chiropractic is based on the idea that all disease is the result of subluxations. It does not agree with the germ theory of disease, and it also rejects the idea of vaccination.

Many chiropractors routinely advise against the vaccination of children. They do not give this advice from a solid medical point of view: it is based on dogmatic adherence to the principles of chiropractic, which has its roots in mysticism and vitalism.

• *Dynamic Thrust.*

This is a Chiropractic adjustment delivered suddenly and forcefully to move vertebrae, often resulting in a "popping" sound. It is usually done without prior warning. This manoeuvre, which may be performed purely for the sound effect, poses a risk of inflicting spinal injury.

• *X-ray overuse.*

Chiropractors use x-rays for diagnostic purposes. Using x-rays in the search for subluxations is believed to have little or no diagnostic value. They are therefore needlessly exposing patients to x-rays: the 24" by 36" full spine x-ray exposing patients to a substantial amount of radiation.

• *Neck manipulation and strokes.*

Neck manipulation is a treatment used by Chiropractors to relieve upper-back pain, headache and migraine suffering.

A Canadian study by the Institute of Clinical Evaluative Sciences in Ontario found that patients younger than 45 who had experienced stroke related to posterior circulation are "5 times more likely than controls to have visited a chiropractor within a week of the event."

Chiropractors admit that neck manipulation can cause strokes; however, they claim that the risk is one in a million. The exact risk is not known, but there is evidence that the likelihood of neck manipulation causing strokes is far higher than the one in a million figure they suggest. . . .

Sudden rotary neck movement, sometimes called "vaster cervical" or "rotary break", is probably the most dangerous practice that Chiropractors perform.

• *Targeting children.*

As with many alternative practitioners, chiropractors are looking to increase their presence in an expanding, lucrative market. One target market seems to be children who, apparently, cannot be too young to have their spines examined and manipulated.

Chiropractors have claimed that conditions that may respond to chiropractic care in babies and young children include: asthma; ear infections; Attention Deficit Disorder; learning disorders; respiratory problems; clumsiness; bed-wetting; stomach problems; hyperactivity; colic; and immune system problems.

Chiropractic has been described as "a treatment in search of a disease". An illustration of this effect was shown when Stephen Barrett, M.D., took a perfectly healthy young girl to five different chiropractors, and each one gave a misdiagnosis based on finding subluxations. This form of subjective diagnosis is common in alternative therapies. Each practitioner coming up with a different diagnosis and treatment to all others practising in exactly the same field.

A claim chiropractors make is that by treating babies and children, they are preventing disease from developing. Proving this type of negative is not possible, and the claim is an emotional appeal to fear.

Paediatricians are qualified doctors who specialise in the treatment of children and many are opposed to so-called Paediatric Chiropractors' claims to be able to cure or prevent childhood illnesses with spinal manipulations. . . .

Chiropractic is a pseudoscientific approach to health care. The thinking behind it has no basis in fact, and even after more than a century, its core belief, the subluxation, cannot be shown to exist, even though it is a scientifically testable theory.

Some of the beliefs, such as the anti-vaccination stance, actually go against scientific evidence, medical opinion and government policy. Opposing germ theory exposes the 19th-century thinking that Chiropractic is based upon.

> "Herbal extracts can be [as] effective [as
> drugs], but are not promoted and are
> highly under-utilized."

Herbal Medicines Are Effective

Danny Siegenthaler

Danny Siegenthaler is an herbalist and an experienced practitioner of Chinese medicine. In the following viewpoint, Siegenthaler argues that herbal medicines have a long history of use in treating ailments. Drug companies recognize this, he states, and have spent a good deal of research time isolating the active ingredients of herbs in order to bottle them and market them. But to keep customers, the pharmaceutical companies must downplay the usefulness of pure herbal remedies even as they plunder these effective natural resources.

As you read, consider the following questions:

1. According to Siegenthaler, what medical properties of dandelions are British scientists investigating?

2. Why does the author think that drug companies' attempts to isolate active ingredients in herbal medicines are wrongheaded?

3. In Siegenthaler's view, why are herbal medicines poor choices for the marketing schemes of drug companies?

Herbs or medicinal plants have a long history in treating disease. In traditional Chinese medicine, for example, the written history of herbal medicine goes back over 2,000 years and herbalists in the West have used "weeds" equally long to treat that which ails us. We are all familiar with the virtues of Garlic, Chamomile, Peppermint, Lavender, and other common herbs.

Interest in medicinal herbs is on the rise again and the interest is primarily from the pharmaceutical industry, which is always looking for 'new drugs' and more effective substances to treat diseases, for which there may be no or very few drugs available.

Considering the very long traditional use of herbal medicines and the large body of evidence of their effectiveness, why is it that we are not generally encouraged to use traditional herbal medicine, instead of synthetic, incomplete copies of herbs, called drugs, considering the millions of dollars being spent looking for these seemingly elusive substances?

Herbs are considered treasures when it comes to ancient cultures and herbalists, and many so-called weeds are worth their weight in gold. Dandelion, Comfrey, Digitalis (Foxglove), the Poppy, Milk Thistle, Stinging Nettle, and many others, have well-researched and established medicinal qualities that have few, if any, rivals in the pharmaceutical industry. Many of them, in fact, form the bases of pharmaceutical drugs.

A Serious Look at Dandelions

Research into the medicinal properties of such herbs as the humble Dandelion is currently being undertaken by scientists at the Royal Botanical Gardens, in Kew, west London, who believe it could be the source of a life-saving drug for cancer patients.

Turmeric, the Wonder Spice

Recently a number of natural compounds—such as resveratrol from red wine and omega-3 fatty acids from fish oil—have begun to receive close scrutiny because preliminary research suggests they might treat and prevent disease inexpensively with few side effects. Turmeric, an orange-yellow powder from an Asian plant, Curcuma longa, has joined this list. No longer is it just an ingredient in vindaloos and tandooris that, since ancient times, has flavored food and prevented spoilage.

A chapter in a forthcoming book, for instance, describes the biologically active components of turmeric—curcumin, and related compounds called curcuminoids—as having antioxidant, anti-inflammatory, antiviral, antibacterial and antifungal properties, with potential activity against cancer, diabetes, arthritis, Alzheimer's disease and other chronic maladies. And in 2005 nearly 300 scientific and technical papers referenced curcumin in the National Library of Medicine's PubMed database, compared with about 100 just five years earlier.

Scientists who sometimes jokingly label themselves curcuminologists are drawn to the compound both because of its many possible valuable effects in the body and its apparent low toxicity. They ponder how the spice or its derivatives might be used, not just as a treatment but as a low-cost preventive medication for some of the most feared ailments.

Gary Stix, "Spice Healer," Scientific American, *vol. 296, no. 2, February 2007, pp. 66–69. www.sciam.com.*

Early tests suggest that it could hold the key to warding off cancer, which kills tens of thousands of people every year.

Their work on the cancer-beating properties of the dandelion, which also has a history of being used to treat warts, is part of a much larger project to examine the natural medicinal properties of scores of British plants and flowers.

Professor Monique Simmonds, head of the Sustainable Uses of Plants Group at Kew, said: "We aren't randomly screening plants for their potential medicinal properties; we are looking at plants which we know have a long history of being used to treat certain medical problems.

"We will be examining them to find out what active compounds they contain which can treat the illness."

Unfortunately, as is so often the case, this group of scientists appears to be looking for active ingredients, which can later be synthesized and then made into pharmaceutical drugs. This is not the way herbs are used traditionally and their functions inevitably change when the active ingredients are used in isolation. That's like saying that the only important part of a car is the engine—nothing else needs to be included.

Looking for the Valuable Ingredient

So, why is there this need for isolating the 'active ingredients'?

As a scientist, I can understand the need for the scientific process of establishing the fact that a particular herb works on a particular disease, pathogen or whatever, and the need to know why and how it does so. But, and this is a BIG but, as a doctor of Chinese medicine I also understand the process of choosing and prescribing *Combinations* of herbs, which have a synergistic effect to treat not just the disease, but any underlying condition as well as the person with the disease. That is a big difference and not one that is easily tested using standard scientific methodologies.

Using anecdotal evidence, which after all has a history of thousands of years, seems to escape my esteemed colleagues all together. Rather than trying to isolate the active ingredient(s), why not test these herbs, utilizing the knowledge of professional herbalists, on patients in vivo, using the myriad of technology available to researchers and medical diagnosticians to see how and why these herbs work in living, breathing patients, rather than in a test tube or on laboratory rats and mice (which, by the way, are not humans and have a different, although somewhat similar, physiology to us)?

I suspect that among the reasons for not following the above procedure is that the pharmaceutical companies are not really interested in the effects of the medicinal plants as a whole, but rather in whether they can isolate a therapeutic substance which can then be manufactured cheaply and marketed as a new drug—and of course that's where the money is.

Herbs Work in Combinations

The problem with this approach is, however, that medicinal plants like Comfrey, Dandelion and other herbs usually contain hundreds if not thousands of chemical compounds that interact, yet many of which are not yet understood and cannot be manufactured. This is why the manufactured drugs, based on so-called active ingredients, often do not work or produce side effects.

Aspirin is a classic case in point. Salicylic acid is the active ingredient in Aspirin tablets, and was first isolated from the bark of the White Willow tree. It is a relatively simple compound to make synthetically, however, Aspirin is known for its ability to cause stomach irritation and in some cases ulceration of the stomach wall.

The herbal extract from the bark of the White Willow tree generally does not cause stomach irritation due to other, so called 'non-active ingredients' contained in the bark, which function to protect the lining of the stomach thereby preventing ulceration of the stomach wall.

Ask yourself, which would I choose: Side effects, or no side effects? It's a very simple answer. Isn't it?

Drug Profiteering

So why then are herbal medicines not used more commonly and why do we have pharmaceutical impostors stuffed down our throats? The answer is, that there's little or no money in herbs for the pharmaceutical companies. They, the herbs, have already been invented, they grow easily, they multiply readily and for the most part, they're freely available.

Furthermore, correctly prescribed and formulated herbal compounds generally resolve the health problem of the patient over a period of time, leaving no requirement to keep taking the preparation—that means no repeat sales. No ongoing prescriptions, no ongoing problem.

Pharmaceuticals, on the other hand, primarily aim to relieve symptoms—that means: ongoing consultations, ongoing sales, ongoing health problems. Which do you think is a more profitable proposition?

Don't get me wrong, this is not to say that all drugs are impostors or that none of the pharmaceutical drugs cure diseases or maladies—they do and some are life-preserving preparations and are without doubt invaluable. However, herbal extracts can be similarly effective, but are not promoted and are highly under-utilized.

Misunderstanding Herbal Remedies

The daily news is full of 'discoveries' of herbs found to be a possible cure of this or that, as in the example of Dandelion and its possible anti-cancer properties. The point is that these herbs need to be investigated in the correct way. They are not just 'an active ingredient'. They mostly have hundreds of ingredients and taking one or two in isolation is not what makes medicinal plants work. In addition, rarely are herbal extracts prescribed by herbalists as singles (a preparation which utilizes only one herb). Usually herbalists mix a variety of medicinal plants to make a mixture, which addresses more than just the major symptoms.

In Chinese medicine, for example, there is a strict order of hierarchy in any herbal prescription, which requires considerable depth of knowledge and experience on the physician's part. The fact that the primary or principle herb has active ingredients, which has a specific physiological effect, does not mean the other herbs are not necessary in the preparation. This is a fact seemingly ignored by the pharmaceutical industry in its need to manufacture new drugs that can control disease.

Knowing that medicinal plants are so effective, that these plants potentially hold the key to many diseases, are inexpensive and have proven their worth time and time again over millennia, why is it that herbal medicine is still not in the forefront of medical treatments, and is considered by many orthodox, medical professionals and pharmaceutical companies as hocus-pocus, hmmm?

> "[T]he consumer has no way to know exactly what is in the [herbal medicine] bottle and what effects the contents may have on health."

Herbal Medicines Vary in Their Effectiveness and Some May Be Dangerous

Jane E. Brody

In the following viewpoint, Jane E. Brody, a health and science reporter for the New York Times, *contends that while some herbal medicines have reported curative properties, many have yielded no documented, beneficial results. A few have even proven toxic. Brody explains that the variety of results has much to do with the lack of regulation and monitoring of herbal medicines, as well as the unstudied long-term consequences of taking such remedies.*

As you read, consider the following questions:

1. What toxins might find their way into herbal medicines, according to Brody?
2. What dangers are posed by Kava and Aristolochia plants, as reported in the viewpoint?

3. As Dr. Stephen E. Strauss explains, why are concise studies of herbal remedies difficult to undertake?

A woman who has been taking a prescription for her high blood pressure was advised by a friend to see an herbalist, who sold her a bag full of remedies. Now, the woman admits, she knows almost nothing about those remedies. Nor has she told her doctor about them.

Are they safe? Are they pure? What drug effects do they have? And what side effects? Will they interact badly with her prescriptions and cause her blood pressure to plunge dangerously low?

She doesn't know, and, chances are, neither does her doctor.

No Assurance of Safety

The woman with high blood pressure is but one of many who wander blindly into the world of herbal remedies, a world that, unlike that of prescription and over-the-counter drugs, remains unregulated. The popularity of these products has soared. In 2001 alone, Americans spent $4.2 billion on herbs and other botanical remedies.

Herbal remedies don't have to meet the standards of safety and purity specified in the Federal Food, Drug and Cosmetic Act. The same applies to vitamins and minerals sold as dietary supplements. And none of them have to be tested to define their medicinal effects.

This is not to say that all these remedies are unsafe, impure or ineffective. Some are made by reputable companies under near-pharmaceutical conditions. Some have been tested in well-designed clinical trials. Still, the consumer has no way to know exactly what is in the bottle and what effects the contents may have on health. Reports of disastrous effects abound, including mania, hemorrhage, coma, heart and kidney damage, liver failure and cancer.

In addition, herbal products may be contaminated with hazardous substances: dangerous plant chemicals, toxic metals, disease-causing micro-organisms, fumigants and pesticides. In some cases, none of them are listed on the label.

Unmonitored Effects

The reported cases of harmful effects represent just a fraction of what actually occurs, since there is no mandated reporting system. Even with prescription and over-the-counter remedies regulated by the government, only an estimated 10 percent of serious adverse effects are ultimately reported to the Food and Drug Administration [FDA], according to an inspector general's report.

With herbal remedies, according to the 1994 Dietary Supplement Health and Education Act, the burden of proof of hazard lies with the FDA, which lacks the resources to monitor these products properly.

Furthermore, only when a hazardous reaction occurs frequently and soon after an herbal remedy is used is the connection likely to be recognized. When ill effects occur infrequently, when they mimic symptoms of an underlying illness or when they develop over time, as liver damage and cancer do, the role of an herbal remedy may be overlooked.

Some herbs are deemed safe because they have been used seemingly safely by herbalists and other traditional healers for centuries.

But as Dr. Peter A. G. M. De Smet of the Netherlands recently stated in the *New England Journal of Medicine*, "If an herb caused an adverse reaction in 1 in 1,000 users, a traditional healer would have to treat 4,800 patients with that herb (i.e., one new patient every single working day for more than 18 years) to have a 95 percent chance of observing the reaction in more than one user."

Kava, long popular for its antianxiety effects, was ultimately found to be toxic to the liver, sometimes damaging it to the point that a transplant is needed. Aristolochia plants have been used for centuries, Dr. De Smet noted, but their ability to cause urothelial cancer has only recently become clear. Likewise, if an herb is toxic to an embryo or fetus, the effect may go unnoticed by a traditional healer, he wrote.

Dr. Stephen E. Straus, director of the National Center for Complementary and Alternative Medicine, wrote in the same journal, "Just because an herb is natural does not mean that it is safe, and claims of remarkable healing powers are rarely supported by evidence."

And, he noted, "With herbal medicines, what is on the label may not be what is in the bottle." In tests of ginseng products he cited, analyses showed that one contained only 12 percent of the amount of active ingredients listed on the label; another contained a whopping 328 percent.

Does Any Herb Work?

Not long ago, nearly half of all prescription drugs were derived from plants or synthesized to mimic a plant chemical. Clearly, plants contain thousands of ingredients with drug effects.

Congress established Dr. Straus's agency to foster studies of the actions and clinical effects of herbal remedies and other alternative medicines and to publicize the findings for doctors and consumers alike.

Studies of herbs, Dr. Straus admits, are not easy to do, in part because it is hard to find standardized sources of herbs, which, unlike manufactured drugs, are by nature complex mixtures of chemicals. Herbal contents can vary based on where, when and how the plants are harvested and how extracts are processed. Researchers cannot be certain which of the many chemicals in an herb contribute to its medicinal effects, if any, or which are harmful.

In his journal review, Dr. De Smet notes that while ginkgo leaf extracts have been promoted for the treatment of demen-

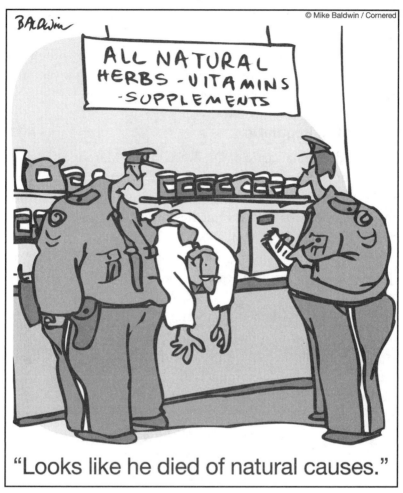

"Cornered," cartoon by Mike Baldwin. CartoonStock.com.

tia, peripheral vascular disease and neurosensory problems like tinnitus, well-designed studies have shown mixed results. The herb may sometimes cause headaches, nausea, gastric symptoms, diarrhea or skin reactions.

Hawthorn appears to improve mild cases of heart failure; saw palmetto improves urinary symptoms in men with benign prostatic enlargement; St. John's wort has helped to relieve mild to moderate depression; feverfew can help to prevent migraine headaches; and ginger can help counteract motion sickness and nausea in pregnancy.

To date, however, the data are inconclusive about the benefits of valerian to counter insomnia, echinacea to prevent and treat common colds and ginseng for any purpose.

Calling for Regulation

In a third journal article, Dr. Donald M. Marcus of Baylor College of Medicine in Houston and Dr. Arthur P. Grollman of the State University of New York at Stony Brook called for new regulations of herbal remedies, which are now subject to lower safety standards than food additives.

They proposed, among other things, requiring the FDA to approve dietary supplements for safety before they can be sold.

They also urged manufacturers to establish and abide by good manufacturing practices and to report all adverse effects promptly to the agency. And they recommended that labels cite all constituents of products by their botanical and common names and list possible harmful effects, including herb-drug interactions.

Further, they suggested establishing expert panels to review the safety of dietary supplements.

Until the regulation of herbal remedies improves, however, it is caveat emptor—let the buyer beware.

Periodical Bibliography

The following articles have been selected to supplement the diverse views presented in this chapter.

Carl E. Bartecchi
"Be Wary of Alternative Medicine," *Denver Business Journal*, January 10, 2003.

Walter A. Brown
"Alternative Medicine: It's Time to Get Smart," *Scientist*, December 7, 1998.

Lorraine Cademartori
"Science vs. Snake Oil," *Forbes*, December 11, 2006.

Consumer Reports
"Alternative Therapies: Beyond the Myths," January 2007.

Edzard Ernst
"Is Homeopathy a Clinically Valuable Approach?" *Trends in Pharmacological Sciences*, November 2006.

Ben Goldacre
"What's Wrong with the Placebo Effect?" *Guardian* (U.K.), April 15, 2004.

Bernadine Healy
"Who Says What's Best?" *U.S. News & World Report*, September 11, 2006.

Ziauddin Sardar
"When Knowledge Is Not the Answer," *New Statesman*, June 12, 2006.

Michael Shermer
"What's the Harm?" *Scientific American*, December 2003.

Jane Spencer
"Alternative-Medicine Usages Holds Risks, WHO Reports," *Wall Street Journal*, June 24, 2004.

Jacob E. Teitelbaum
"Why Bother with Natural Therapies," *Total Health*, March 2006.

Kakkib li'Dthia Warrawee'a
"Wisdom, Knowledge, and Information: Have We Lost Our Way in Our Understanding and Practice of Medicine?" *Journal of Alternative and Complementary Medicine*, 2004.

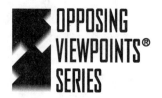OPPOSING
VIEWPOINTS®
SERIES

CHAPTER 2

Why Is Alternative Medicine Popular?

Chapter Preface

In a 2005 article that appeared in the *Medical Journal of Australia*, Wallace Sampson and Kimball Atwood IV, two American medical professionals, argue that the nature of the postmodern world has bred a tolerance for absurdity that in turn has made complementary and alternative medicine (CAM) both legitimate and popular. In Sampson and Atwood's view, postmodernism has undermined hierarchies and made all sources of knowledge and theoretical speculation equally valid. In terms of health care, this has meant that conventional medicine is no longer the one, objective pathway to healing, but rather one among many health philosophies. Accordingly, each philosophy is welcomed into the plurality of diverse healing arts, or as Sampson and Atwood contend, "Various 'schools' and philosophies of healing—each inconsistent with the others, such as chiropractic, homoeopathy, orthomolecular medicine, and traditional Chinese medicine—create a scientific multiculturalism" in which "implausible proposals and claims become tolerable and comfortable."

Sampson and Atwood maintain that clinical trials and evidence gained from scientific inquiry and experimentation should cut short this trend in postmodern thinking and reveal the absurdity of unproven, ineffectual therapies. However, the authors state that because evidence-based medicine has no solid testing criteria and that results of trials are often inconsistent, complementary and alternative medicine has claimed that its own inconsistencies are not proof of ineffectiveness. Therefore, Sampson and Atwood attest that "most CAM systems remain in an indeterminate limbo state, awaiting enough negative clinical trials to return consensus opinion to the state of decades prior."

Sampson and Atwood use their argument to explain the popularity of CAM by showing how, in their opinion, absurd thinking has achieved respectability in a society that chooses not to criticize ways of thinking even if they are faulty or not based on observable fact. Once enough people accept alternative medicine, the authors believe, it becomes legitimized— not by scientific trial, but by its place in the economy, in pop culture, and in the medical institutions that continually fund its research. And once it achieves a hint of validation, more people become willing experimenters and potential advocates of its wider use.

The authors of the viewpoints in the following chapter offer other opinions on why alternative medicine is so popular today. While not all of the authors are critics in the vein of Sampson and Atwood, the majority note that people's faith in complementary and alternative medicine has much to do with their willingness to accept its usefulness and their lack of trust that conventional medicine can provide all the answers.

| *"In ways large and small, millions of people are taking active steps to venture outside the mainstream. . . ."*

People Choose Alternative Medicine Because They Are Dissatisfied with Conventional Medicine

Benedict Carey

In the following viewpoint, Benedict Carey, a health writer for the New York Times, *reports that many Americans are turning to alternative medicine because of their dissatisfaction with conventional medicine. As Carey relates, these people are typically outraged at conventional healthcare costs, disappointed with impersonal doctors, and displeased by the side-effects of prescription drugs. They believe alternative medicine offers more individualized care over which they have more control.*

As you read, consider the following questions:

1. According to Carey, what patients are least likely to experiment with alternative therapies?

2. As reported in the viewpoint, what did a naturopath prescribe to Cynthia Riley to counter her diagnosed reaction to metal exposure?

3. In Carey's view, what is "the sentiment that many Americans say they feel is missing from conventional medicine?"

A few moments before boarding a plane from Los Angeles to New York in January, Charlene Solomon performed her usual preflight ritual: she chewed a small tablet that contained trace amounts of several herbs, including extracts from daisy and chamomile plants.

Ms. Solomon, 56, said she had no way to know whether the tablet, an herb-based remedy for jet lag, worked as advertised. Researchers have found no evidence that such preparations are effective, and Ms. Solomon knows that most doctors would scoff that she was wasting her money.

Yet she swears by the tablets, as well as other alternative remedies, for reasons she acknowledges are partly psychological.

"I guess I do believe in the power of simply paying attention to your health, which in a way is what I'm doing," said Ms. Solomon, who runs a Web consulting business in Los Angeles. "But I also believe there are simply a lot of unknowns when it comes to staying healthy, and if there's a possibility something will help I'm willing to try it."

Besides, she added, "whatever I'm doing is working, so I'm going to keep doing it."

Showing Loyalty to Alternative Medicine

The most telling evidence of Americans' dissatisfaction with traditional health care is the more than $27 billion they spend annually on alternative and complementary medicine, according to government estimates. In ways large and small, millions of people are taking active steps to venture outside the mainstream, whether by taking the herbal remedy echinacea for a cold or by placing their last hopes for cancer cure in alternative treatment, as did Coretta Scott King, who died [in February 2006] at an alternative hospice clinic in Mexico.

They do not appear to care that there is little, if any, evidence that many of the therapies work. Nor do they seem to mind that alternative therapy practitioners have a fraction of the training mainstream doctors do or that vitamin and herb makers are as profit-driven as drug makers.

This straying from conventional medicine is often rooted in a sense of disappointment, even betrayal, many patients and experts say. When patients see conventional medicine's inadequacies up close—a misdiagnosis, an intolerable drug, failed surgery, even a dismissive doctor—many find the experience profoundly disillusioning, or at least eye-opening.

Haggles with insurance providers, conflicting findings from medical studies and news reports of drug makers' covering up product side effects all feed their disaffection, to the point where many people begin to question not only the health care system but also the science behind it. Soon, intuition and the personal experience of friends and family may seem as trustworthy as advice from a doctor in diagnosing an illness or judging a treatment.

What Is Appealing about Alternative Medicine

Experts say that people with serious medical problems like diabetes or cancer are least likely to take their chances with natural medicine, unless their illness is terminal. Consumers generally know that quackery is widespread in alternative practices, that there is virtually no government oversight of so-called natural remedies and that some treatments, like enemas, can be dangerous.

Still, 48 percent of American adults used at least one alternative or complementary therapy in 2004, up from 42 percent a decade ago, a figure that includes students and retirees, soccer moms and truckers, New Age seekers and religious conservatives. The numbers continue to grow, experts say, for reasons that have as much to do with increasing distrust of mainstream medicine and the psychological appeal of nontraditional approaches as with the therapeutic properties of herbs or other supplements.

"I think there is a powerful element of nostalgia at work for many people, for home remedies—for what healing is supposed to be—combined with an idealized vision of what is natural and whole and good," said Dr. Linda Barnes, a medical anthropologist at Boston University School of Medicine.

Dr. Barnes added, "People look around and feel that the conventional system does not measure up, and that something deeper about their well-being is not being addressed at all."

Taking Responsibility for One's Health

Ms. Solomon's first small steps outside the mainstream came in 1991, after she watched her mother die of complications from a hysterectomy.

"I saw doctors struggling to save her," she said. "They were trying really hard, and I have great respect for what they do, but at that point I realized the doctors could only do so much."

She decided then that she needed to take more responsibility for her own health, by eating better, exercising more and seeking out health aids that she thought of as natural, meaning not prescribed by a doctor or developed by a pharmaceutical company.

"I usually stay away from drugs if I can, because the side effects even of cough and cold medicines can be pretty strong," she said.

The herbal preparations she uses, she said, "have no side effects, and the difference in my view is that they help support my own body's natural capability, to fight off disease" rather than treat symptoms.

If these sentiments are present in someone like Ms. Solomon, who regularly consults her internist and describes herself as "pretty mainstream," they run far deeper in millions of other people who use nontraditional therapies more often.

In interviews and surveys, these patients often described prescription drugs as poisons that mostly mask symptoms without improving their underlying cause.

Many extend their suspicions further. In a 2004 study, researchers at the University of Arizona conducted interviews with a group of men and women in Tucson who suffered from chronic arthritis, most of whom regularly used alternative therapies. Those who used alternative methods exclusively valued the treatments on the "rightness of fit" above other factors, and they were inherently skeptical of the health care system.

Adverse to Drug Companies

Distrust in the medical industrial complex, as some patients call it, stems in part from suspicions that insurers warp medical decision making, and in part from the belief that drug companies are out to sell as many drugs as possible, regardless of patients' needs, interviews show.

"I do partly blame the drug companies and the money they make" for the breakdown in trust in the medical system, said Joyce Newman, 74, of Lynnwood, Wash., who sees a natural medicine specialist as her primary doctor. "The time when you would listen to your doctor and do whatever he said—that time is long gone, in my opinion. You have to learn to use your own head."

From here it is a small step to begin doubting medical science. If Western medicine is imperfect and sometimes corrupt, then mainstream doctors may not be the best judge of treatments after all, many patients conclude. People's actual experience—the personal testimony of friends and family, in particular—feels more truthful.

To best way to validate this, said Ms. Newman and many others who regularly use nontraditional therapies, is simply to try a remedy "and listen to your own body."

Ignored by Conventional Doctors

Cynthia Riley effectively opted out of mainstream medicine when it seemed that doctors were not listening to her.

During a nine-year period that ended in 2004, Ms. Riley, 47, visited almost 20 doctors, for a variety of intermittent and strange health complaints: blurred vision, urinary difficulties, balance problems so severe that at times she wobbled like a drunk.

She felt unwell most of the time, but doctors could not figure out what she had.

Each specialist ordered different tests, depending on the symptom, Ms. Riley said, but they were usually rushed and seemed to solicit her views only as a formality.

Undeterred, Ms. Riley, an event planner who lives near New London, Conn., typed out a four-page description of her ordeal, including her suspicion that she suffered from lead poisoning. One neurologist waved the report away as if insulted; another barely skimmed it, she said.

"I remember sitting in one doctor's office and realizing, 'He thinks I'm crazy,'" Ms. Riley said. "I was getting absolutely nowhere in conventional medicine, and I was determined to get to the root of my problems."

Through word of mouth, Ms. Riley heard about Deirdre O'Connor, a naturopath with a thriving practice in nearby Mystic, Conn., and made an appointment.

In recent years, people searching for something outside of conventional medicine have increasingly turned to naturopaths, herbal specialists who must complete a degree that includes some standard medical training in order to be licensed, experts say. Fourteen states, including California and Connecticut, now license naturopaths to practice medicine. Natu-

Impersonalized Health Care

When today's doctors do talk about the problems of life with their patients, they usually have at least one eye on the diagnostic categories of mental illness. Rather than exploring life's issues philosophically, doctors wonder whether a whining patient has a form of depression that needs to be treated with medication. Thus, even the management of emotional trouble becomes rather cookbook. The doctor becomes a skilled tradesman, such as a plumber or electrician—someone whose work calls for little depth of human understanding.

Patients see this, and they are repelled by it. This is one reason they flock to alternative medicine. While alternative medicine encompasses different treatment modalities, most of these systems have something in common: They do not herd patients into diagnostic categories or cause patients to be managed according to some predetermined algorithm. Each patient is considered unique in alternative medicine, such that if 10 patients present to an acupuncturist with peptic ulcer disease, each one might be treated differently.

Ronald W. Dworkin,
"Science, Faith, and Alternative Medicine,"
Policy Review, *August–September 2001.*
www.hoover.org/publications/policyreview.

ral medicine groups are pushing for similar legislation in other states, including New York.

Licensed naturopaths can prescribe drugs from an approved list in some states, but have no prescribing rights in others.

Right away, Ms. Riley said, she noticed a difference in the level of service. Before even visiting the office, she received a fat envelope in the mail containing a four-page questionnaire, she said. In addition to asking detailed questions about medical history—standard information—it asked about energy level, foods she craved, sensitivity to weather and self-image: "Please list adjectives that describe you," read one item.

"It felt right, from the beginning," Ms. Riley said.

Feeling Better

Her first visit lasted an hour and a half, and Ms. O'Connor, the naturopath, agreed that metal exposure was a possible cause of her symptoms. It emerged in their interview that Ms. Riley had worked in the steel industry, and tests of her hair and urine showed elevated levels of both lead and mercury, Ms. O'Connor said.

After taking a combination of herbs, vitamins and regular doses of a drug called dimercaptosuccinic acid, or DMSA, to treat lead poisoning, Ms. Riley said, she began to feel better, and the symptoms subsided.

Along the way, Ms. O'Connor explained the treatments to Ms. Riley, sometimes using drawings, and called her patient regularly to check in, especially during the first few months, Ms. Riley said.

Other doctors said they could not comment on Ms. Riley's case because they had not examined her. Researchers who specialize in lead poisoning say that it is rare in adults but that it can cause neurological symptoms and bladder problems and is often missed by primary care doctors.

Dr. Herbert Needleman, a psychiatrist who directs the lead research group at the University of Pittsburgh, said DMSA was the pharmaceutical treatment of choice for high blood lead levels.

Researchers say there is little or no evidence that vitamins or herbs can relieve symptoms like Ms. Riley's. Still, she said, "I look and feel better than I have in years."

Life and Death

Diane Paradise bet her life on the uncertain benefits of natural medicine, after being burned physically and emotionally by conventional doctors.

In 1995, doctors told Ms. Paradise, now 35, that she had Hodgkin's disease. After a six-month course of chemotherapy and radiation, she said, she was declared cancer free, and she remained healthy for five years.

But in 2001 the cancer reappeared, more advanced, and her doctors recommended a 10-month course of drugs and radiation, plus a marrow transplant, she said.

Ms. Paradise, a marketing consultant in Rochester, N.Y., balked.

"I was burned badly the first time around, third-degree burns, and now they were talking about 10 months," she said in an interview, "and they were giving me no guarantees; they said it was experimental. That's when I started looking around. I really had nothing to lose, and I was focused on quality of life at that point, not quantity."

When she told one of her doctors that she was considering an alternative treatment in Arizona, the man exploded, she said.

"His exact words were, 'That's not treatment, that's a vacation—you're wasting your time!'" she said.

And so ended the relationship. With help from friends, Ms. Paradise raised about $40,000 to pay for the Arizona clinic's treatment, plus living expenses while there.

"I had absolutely no scientific reason for choosing this route, none," she said. "I just think there are times in our life when we are asked to make decisions based on our intuition, on our gut instinct, not based on evidence put in front of us, and for me this was one of those moments."

Cancer researchers say that there is no evidence that vitamins, herbs or other alternative therapies can cure cancer, and they caution that some regimens may worsen the disease.

But Ms. Paradise said that her relationship with the natural medicine specialist in Arizona had been collaborative and that she had felt "more empowered, more involved" in the treatment plan, which included large doses of vitamins, as well as changes in diet and sleep routines. After four months on the regimen, she said, she felt much better.

But the cancer was not cured. It has resurfaced recently [as of 2006] and spread, and this time Ms. Paradise has started an experimental treatment with an oncologist in New York.

She is complementing this treatment, she said, with another course of alternative therapy in Arizona. She moved in with friends near Phoenix and started the alternative regime in January.

"It's 79 degrees and beautiful here," she said by phone in mid-January. "Let's hope that's a good sign."

Something Missing in Conventional Medicine

For all their suspicions and questions about conventional medicine, those who venture outside the mainstream tend to have one thing in abundance, experts say: hope. In a 1998 survey of more than 1,000 adults from around the country, researchers found that having an interest in "personal growth or spirituality" predicted alternative medicine use.

Nontraditional healers know this, and they often offer some spiritual element in their practice, if they think it is appropriate. David Wood, a naturopath who with his wife, Cheryl, runs a large, Christian-oriented practice in Lynnwood, Wash., said he treated patients of all faiths.

"We pray with patients, with their permission," said Mr. Wood, who also works with local medical doctors when necessary. "If patients would not like us to pray for them, we don't, but it's there if needed."

He added, "Our goal here is to help people get really well, not merely free of symptoms."

That is exactly the sentiment that many Americans say they feel is missing from conventional medicine. Whatever the benefits and risks of its many concoctions and methods, alternative medicine offers them at least the promise of affectionate care, unhurried service, freedom from prescription drug side effects and the potential for feeling not just better but also spiritually recharged.

"I don't hate doctors or anything," Ms. Newman said. "I just know they can make mistakes, and so often they refer you on to see another doctor, and another."

Seeing a naturopath, she said, "I feel I'm known, they see me as a whole person, they listen to what I say."

> "Science may not have all the answers, but quackery has no answers at all! It will take your money and break your heart."

People Choose Alternative Medicine Because They Fall for Sales Pitches

Stephen Barrett and William Jarvis

In the following viewpoint, Stephen Barrett and William T. Jarvis argue that the promoters and sellers of alternative medicine use many tricks to convince people to use their products and treatments. The authors state that alternative medicine purveyors appeal to consumer's fears and hopes, capitalizing on their dissatisfaction with conventional medicine and their desire to have more control over their healthcare. To reinforce these notions, marketers suggest that alternative therapies offer a means to move beyond the limitations of conventional medicine.

As you read, consider the following questions:

1. Why are testimonials the "cornerstone" of alternative medicine's sales success, according to Barrett and Jarvis?

Stephen Barrett and William Jarvis, "How Quackery Sells," *www.quackwatch.org*, January 20, 2005. Reproduced by permission.

2. In the authors' view, why is deception of the terminally ill "the cruelest form of quackery"?

3. As the authors state, how do alternative medicine promoters use "conspiracy" theories to help market their products?

Modern health quacks are supersalesmen. They play on fear. They cater to hope. And once they have you, they'll keep you coming back for more . . . and more . . . and more. Seldom do their victims realize how often or how skillfully they are cheated. Does the mother who feels good as she hands her child a vitamin think to ask herself whether he really needs it? Do subscribers to "health food" publications realize that articles are slanted to stimulate business for their advertisers? Not usually.

Most people think that quackery is easy to spot. Often it is not. Its promoters wear the cloak of science. They use scientific terms and quote (or misquote) scientific references. Talk show hosts may refer to them as experts or as "scientists ahead of their time." The very word "quack" helps their camouflage by making us think of an outlandish character selling snake oil from the back of a covered wagon—and, of course, no intelligent people would buy snake oil nowadays, would they?

Well, maybe snake oil isn't selling so well, lately. But acupuncture? "Organic" foods? Hair analysis? The latest diet book? Megavitamins? "Stress formulas"? Cholesterol-lowering teas? Homeopathic remedies? Magnets? Nutritional "cures" for AIDS? Products that "cleanse your system"? Or shots to pep you up? Business is booming for health quacks. Their annual take is in the *billions!* Spot reducers, "immune boosters," water purifiers, "ergogenic aids," systems to "balance body chemistry," special diets for arthritis. Their product list is endless.

What sells is not the quality of their products, but their ability to influence their audience. To those in pain, they promise relief. To the incurable, they offer hope. To the nutrition-conscious, they say, "Make sure you have enough." To a public worried about pollution, they say, "Buy natural." To one and all, they promise better health and a longer life. Modern quacks can reach people emotionally.

Appeals to Vanity

An attractive young airline stewardess once told a physician that she was taking more than 20 vitamin pills a day. "I used to feel run-down all the time," she said, "but now I feel really great!"

"Yes," the doctor replied, "but there is no scientific evidence that extra vitamins can do that. Why not take the pills one month on, one month off, to see whether they really help you or whether it's just a coincidence. After all, $300 a year is a lot of money to be wasting."

"Look, doctor," she said. "I don't care what you say. I KNOW the pills are helping me."

How was this bright young lady converted into a true believer? First, an appeal to her curiosity persuaded her to try and see. Then an appeal to her vanity convinced her to disregard scientific evidence in favor of personal experience—to think for herself. Supplementation is encouraged by a distorted concept of biochemical individuality—that everyone is unique enough to disregard the Recommended Dietary Allowances (RDAs). Quacks won't tell you that scientists deliberately set the RDAs high enough to allow for individual differences. A more dangerous appeal of this type is the suggestion that although a remedy for a serious disease has not been shown to work for other people, it still might work for you. (You are extraordinary!)

A more subtle appeal to your vanity underlies the message of the TV ad quack: Do it yourself—be your own doctor. "Anyone out there have 'tired blood'?" he used to wonder (Don't bother to find out what's wrong with you, however. Just try my tonic.) "Troubled with irregularity?" he asks. (Pay no attention to the doctors who say you don't need a daily movement. Just use my laxative.) "Want to kill germs on contact?" (Never mind that mouthwash doesn't prevent colds.) "Trouble sleeping?" (Don't bother to solve the underlying problem. Just try my sedative.)

Turning Customers into Salespeople

Most people who think they have been helped by an unorthodox method enjoy sharing their success stories with their friends. People who give such testimonials are usually motivated by a sincere wish to help their fellow humans. Rarely do they realize how difficult it is to evaluate a "health" product on the basis of personal experience. Like the airline stewardess, the average person who feels better after taking a product will not be able to rule out coincidence (spontaneous remission)—or the placebo effect (feeling better because he thinks he has taken a positive step). Since we tend to believe what others tell us of personal experiences, testimonials can be powerful persuaders. Despite their unreliability, they are the cornerstone of the quack's success.

Multilevel companies that sell nutritional products systematically turn their customers into salespeople. "When you share our products," says the sales manual of one such company, "you're not just selling. You're passing on news about products you believe in to people you care about. Make a list of people you know; you'll be surprised how long it will be. This list is your first source of potential customers." A sales leader from another company suggests, "Answer all objections with testimonials. That's the secret to motivating people!"...

The Use of Fear

The sale of vitamins has become so profitable that some otherwise reputable manufacturers are promoting them with misleading claims. For example, for many years, Lederle Laboratories (makers of *Stresstabs*) and Hoffmann-La Roche advertised in major magazines that stress "robs" the body of vitamins and creates significant danger of vitamin deficiencies.

Another slick way for quackery to attract customers is the invented disease. Virtually everyone has symptoms of one sort or another—minor aches or pains, reactions to stress or hormone variations, effects of aging, etc. Labeling these ups and downs of life as symptoms of disease enables the quack to provide "treatment."

Some practitioners claim to detect "deficiencies" (or "imbalances" or "toxins," etc.) before any symptoms appear or before they can be detected by conventional means. Then they can sell you supplements (or balance you, or remove toxins, etc.). And when the terrible consequences they warn about don't develop, they can claim success. . . .

Hope for Sale

Since ancient times, people have sought at least four different magic potions: the love potion, the fountain of youth, the cure-all, and the athletic superpill. Quackery has always been willing to cater to these desires. It used to offer unicorn horn, special elixirs, amulets, and magical brews. Today's products are vitamins, bee pollen, ginseng, Gerovital, pyramids, "glandular extracts," biorhythm charts, aromatherapy, and many more. Even reputable products are promoted as though they are potions. Toothpastes and colognes will improve our love life. Hair preparations and skin products will make us look "younger than our years." Olympic athletes tell us that breakfast cereals will make us champions. And youthful models reassure us that cigarette smokers are sexy and have fun.

False hope for the seriously ill is the cruelest form of quackery because it can lure victims away from effective treatment. Even when death is inevitable, however, false hope can do great damage. Experts who study the dying process tell us that while the initial reaction is shock and disbelief, most terminally ill patients will adjust very well as long as they do not

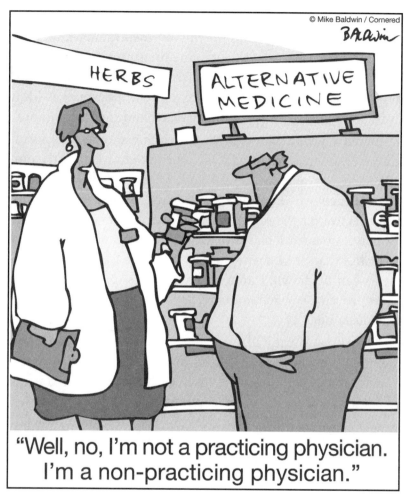

"Cornered," cartoon by Mike Baldwin. CartoonStock.com.

feel abandoned. People who accept the reality of their fate not only die psychologically prepared, but also can put their affairs in order. On the other hand, those who buy false hope can get stuck in an attitude of denial. They waste not only financial resources but what little remaining time they have left.

Clinical Tricks

The most important characteristic to which the success of quacks can be attributed is probably their ability to exude confidence. Even when they admit that a method is unproven, they can attempt to minimize this by mentioning how difficult and expensive it is to get something proven to the satisfaction of the FDA [Food and Drug Administration] these days. If they exude self-confidence and enthusiasm, it is likely to be contagious and spread to patients and their loved ones.

Because people like the idea of making choices, quacks often refer to their methods as "alternatives." Correctly employed, it can refer to aspirin and Tylenol as alternatives for the treatment of minor aches and pains. Both are proven safe and effective for the same purpose. Lumpectomy can be an alternative to radical mastectomy for breast cancer. Both have verifiable records of safety and effectiveness from which judgments can be drawn. Can a method that is unsafe, ineffective, or unproven be a genuine alternative to one that is proven? Obviously not. . . .

Quacks also capitalize on the natural healing powers of the body by taking credit whenever possible for improvement in a patient's condition. One multilevel company—anxious to avoid legal difficulty in marketing its herbal concoction— makes no health claims whatsoever. "You take the product," a spokesperson suggests on the company's introductory videotape, "and tell me what it does for you." An opposite tack— shifting blame—is used by many cancer quacks. If their treatment doesn't work, it's because radiation and/or chemotherapy have "knocked out the immune system."

Another selling trick is the use of weasel words. Quacks often use this technique in suggesting that one or more items on a list is reason to suspect that you *may* have a vitamin deficiency, a yeast infection, or whatever else they are offering to fix.

The disclaimer is a related tactic. Instead of promising to cure your specific disease, some quacks will offer to "cleanse" or "detoxify" your body, balance its chemistry, release its "nerve energy," bring it in harmony with nature, or do other things to "help the body to heal itself." This type of disclaimer serves two purposes. Since it is impossible to measure the processes the quack describes, it is difficult to prove him wrong. In addition, if the quack is not a physician, the use of nonmedical terminology may help to avoid prosecution for practicing medicine without a license. . . .

Another potent technique is cultural association, in which promoters ally themselves with religious or other cultural beliefs by associating their product or service with an article of faith or prejudice of their target audience.

In a contest for patient satisfaction, art will beat science nearly every time. Quacks are masters at the art of delivering health care. The secret to this art is to make the patient believe that he is cared about as a person. To do this, quacks lather love lavishly. One way this is done is by having receptionists make notes on the patients' interests and concerns in order to recall them during future visits. This makes each patient feel special in a very personal sort of way. Some quacks even send birthday cards to every patient. Although seductive tactics may give patients a powerful psychological lift, they may also encourage over-reliance on an inappropriate therapy. . . .

Handling the Opposition

Quacks are involved in a constant struggle with legitimate health care providers, mainstream scientists, government regulatory agencies and consumer protection groups. Despite the strength of this science-based opposition, quackery manages to flourish. To maintain their credibility, quacks use a variety of clever propaganda ploys. Here are some favorites:

"They persecuted Galileo!" The history of science is laced with instances where great pioneers and their discoveries were met with resistance. Harvey (nature of blood circulation), Lister (antiseptic technique) and Pasteur (germ theory) are notable examples. Today's quack boldly asserts that he is another example of someone ahead of his time. Close examination, however, will show how unlikely this is. First of all, the early pioneers who were persecuted lived during times that were much less scientific. In some cases, opposition to their ideas stemmed from religious forces. Secondly, it is a basic principle of the scientific method that the burden of proof belongs to the proponent of a claim. The ideas of Galileo, Harvey, Lister and Pasteur overcame their opposition because their soundness can be demonstrated.

A related ploy, which is a favorite with cancer quacks, is the charge of "conspiracy." How can we be sure that the AMA [American Medical Association], the FDA, the American Cancer Society, drug companies and others are not involved in some monstrous plot to withhold a cancer cure from the public? To begin with, history reveals no such practice in the past. The elimination of serious diseases is not a threat to the medical profession—doctors prosper by curing diseases, not by keeping people sick. It should also be apparent that modern medical technology has not altered the zeal of scientists to eliminate disease. When polio was conquered, iron lungs became virtually obsolete, but nobody resisted this advancement because it would force hospitals to change. Neither will medical scientists mourn the eventual defeat of cancer. Moreover, how could a conspiracy to withhold a cancer cure hope to be successful? Many physicians die of cancer each year. Do you believe that the vast majority of doctors would conspire to withhold a cure for a disease which affects them, their colleagues and their loved ones? To be effective, a conspiracy would have to be worldwide. If laetrile, for example, really worked, many other nations' scientists would soon realize it. . . .

Quacks like to charge that, "Science doesn't have all the answers." That's true, but it doesn't claim to have them. Rather, it is a rational and responsible process that can answer many questions—including whether procedures are safe and effective for their intended purpose. It is quackery that constantly claims to have answers for incurable diseases. The idea that people should turn to quack remedies when frustrated by science's inability to control a disease is irrational. Science may not have all the answers, but quackery has no answers at all! It will take your money and break your heart.

Many treatments advanced by the scientific community are later shown to be unsafe or worthless. Doctors also make mistakes. Such failures become grist for organized quackery's public relations mill in its ongoing attack on science. Actually, "failures" reflect a key element of science: its willingness to test its methods and beliefs and abandon those shown to be invalid. True medical scientists have no philosophical commitment to particular treatment approaches, only a commitment to develop and use methods that are safe and effective for an intended purpose. When a quack remedy flunks a scientific test, its proponents merely reject the test. . . .

How to Avoid Being Tricked

The best way to avoid being tricked is to stay away from tricksters. Unfortunately, in health matters, this is no simple task. Quackery is not sold with a warning label. Moreover, the dividing line between what is quackery and what is not is by no means sharp. A product that is effective in one situation may be part of a quack scheme in another. (Quackery lies in the promise, not the product.) Practitioners who use effective methods may also use ineffective ones. For example, they may mix valuable advice to stop smoking with unsound advice to take vitamins. Even outright quacks may relieve some psychosomatic ailments with their reassuring manner.

| *"Homeopathy and the others can only work as long as their myths and meanings survive. . . ."*

People Choose Alternative Medicine Because They Want to Believe It Works

Ben Goldacre

Ben Goldacre is a journalist and doctor who writes the "Bad Science" column for the Guardian, *a major British newspaper. In the following viewpoint, Goldacre discusses the placebo effect, a medical phenomenon through which patients accept the efficacy of medicines because they want to believe that they work. Goldacre says that alternative medicines and treatments function in this manner because none have been proven to be scientifically effective. However, placebos do have a psychological effect, Goldacre maintains, and because people choose to believe in the placebo effects of alternative therapies, these practices will likely persist.*

As you read, consider the following questions:

1. Why does Goldacre say that placebo is "the most interesting phenomenon in medicine"?

2. How does "branding" help sell efficacy in medicines, as Goldacre explains?

3. To Goldacre, what has conventional medicine "championed" in place of paternalism?

Sceptics, and the placebo effect, are easily misunderstood. Since I've made a modest second career out of rubbishing alternative therapies (or rather the pseudoscience of the claims behind them), you might expect me to be pleased with a new analysis of 110 placebo-controlled randomised trials of homoeopathy, published in the *Lancet* [a British medical journal], showing there is no evidence that homeopathic tablets perform any better than placebos. Obviously, it's an important and useful finding. But it misses the mark.

The placebo is arguably the most interesting phenomenon in medicine, because it goes far beyond the effectiveness of little white sugar pills, into the cultural meaning of treatment. It has been shown, for example, that green sugar pills are a more effective treatment for anxiety than red sugar pills, because of the cultural meaning, we might parsimoniously assume, of the colours green and red.

Likewise, studies have found that salt-water injections can be a more effective placebo treatment than white sugar pills— not, I might add, because there is anything particularly useful about salt water injections, but because the ceremony of performing an injection is a far more invasive, authoritative and dramatic intervention.

It gets far stranger. A placebo operation in the 1950s was found to be as effective for the treatment of angina as the real operation it was being compared with. Reading the paper 50 years later, the most striking part is the discussion section, where they quietly drop the operation and nobody stands up to point out the incredibly strange discovery that a placebo operation works for anything, let alone angina.

Sham Surgery

Forty years ago, a young Seattle cardiologist named Leonard Cobb conducted a unique trial of a procedure then commonly used for angina, in which doctors made small incisions in the chest and tied knots in two arteries to try to increase blood flow to the heart. It was a popular technique—90 percent of patients reported that it helped— but when Cobb compared it with placebo surgery in which he made incisions but did not tie off the arteries, the sham operations proved just as successful. The procedure, known as internal mammary ligation, was soon abandoned. Over the next decades, the whole idea of placebo surgery fell out of favor with ethicists and patient advocates. . . .

Some doctors argue, with reason, that the new enthusiasm for placebo surgery is driven by hospital bean counters and insurers who want hard evidence that an expensive procedure works before they'll pay for it. And yet, with all due respect for medical economics, that can't be the only explanation. If placebo surgery makes sense, it makes sense because of the growing body of evidence for the strength of the placebo effect in general. Maybe pretend operations are just the most sensational proof of a diffuse phenomenon that has never quite been explained, but that, as the historian of science Anne Harrington has written, continues to "haunt our house of biomedical objectivity."

Margaret Talbot, "The Placebo Prescription,"
New York Times, *January 9, 2000. www.nytimes.com.*

Engineering the Idea of Efficacy

Branding, of course, is the key to the efficacy of little white sugar pills. Marketing, after all, is nothing if not engineered cultural meaning. A four-way comparison among sugar pills and aspirin, in either unbranded aspirin boxes or packaging mocked up to look like the Disprin brand, showed that the brand-name packaging works, because of the huge wealth of cultural background material—the adverts, the word-of-mouth endorsement, the childhood experiences—that packaging plays on. The change in packaging had almost as big an impact on pain as whether the pills actually had any drug in them.

The implication for rationalists, who reach for generic, un-branded medications like aspirin and ibuprofen in preference to Disprin or Nurofen, is clear. It's perfectly rational to believe that expensive Nurofen is more effective than cheap un-branded ibuprofen, even if they've both got the same active ingredient—but only, in a peculiar tautology, if that's what you believe.

This, of course, is the key also to alternative medicine: ho-meopathy is what you might call a "complex intervention", rich in cultural meaning and drawing on such attractive con-temporary ideas as individualism, patient empowerment and personalised healthcare. But all alternative therapies also offer something very much missing from modern medicine, the idea of containment of symptoms.

Transparent modern medics often say: "I don't know what the cause of your problem is. This might make it better, but it might not, and it might have these side effects." They some-times follow this with: "What do you think?"

Enter the alternative therapist, who understands your problems whatever they are, who is privately employed and has time to listen, who has an answer and who gives a compli-cated (often wilfully obscure but always authoritative) expla-nation of what is going on, maintaining the power imbalance in the therapeutic relationship with his or her exclusive access to arcane knowledge. If that's not old-fashioned medical pa-ternalism, I don't know what is, and the paradox is clear: while modern medicine, without even pausing to discuss the question, has championed patient autonomy and informed consent—and thrown the placebo effect out of the window—

the market has shown that the old paternalism, in a new guise, is still very popular.

The Trappings of Cultural Meaning

Whether mainstream medics would want to go back to the old ways and embrace the placebo-maximising wiles of the alternative therapists is an easy question: no thanks. The didactic, paternalistic, authoritative, mystifying mantle has passed to the alternative therapist, and to wear it requires one thing most doctors are uncomfortable with, dishonesty.

So the fact stands, not even slightly mocking us, that in many cases homeopathy does seem to help, as a complex intervention, laden with branded cultural meaning, at least better than "doing nothing". It is no better than placebo, because it is placebo, in all its rich glory.

But the homeopaths themselves can never admit this clear, compelling, evidence-based and parsimonious explanation: they need the memory of water, the power of arcane knowledge and all the rest. Homeopathy and the others can only work as long as their myths and meanings survive, and so medics, alternative therapists—and smarmy sceptics—will always, mercifully, be in business.

> "Growing national interest in comple-
> mentary and alternative medicine
> therapies provides an opportunity for
> employers to rethink the way they ap-
> proach health benefits."

Employers Choose Alternative Medicine to Combat Health Care Costs

George DeVries

George DeVries states in the following viewpoint that many American businesses are offering employees health coverage for alternative medicine. As DeVries notes, these employers have decided to include alternative care health benefits in response to studies that show that employees who use alternative therapies as part of preventative medical care have reduced serious health-care visits and consequently lowered employer expenses. Other research has suggested that alternative treatments—such as massage and yoga—also reduce job stress and increase worker productivity, DeVries writes. DeVries is president of American Spe-

George DeVries, "Using Complementary and Alternative Medicine Insurance to Contain Health Care Costs," *Benefits and Compensation Digest*, September 2006, pp. 20–22. Reproduced with permission from the Benefits and Compensation Digest, Volume 43, No. 9, published by the International Foundation of Employee Benefit Plans (www.ifebp.org), Brookfield, WI.

cialty Health, a San Diego company that conducts employee wellness programs and markets alternative healthcare products.

As you read, consider the following questions:

1. According to the cited 2006 Deloitte & Touche survey, what percentage of American employers had implemented programs to aid employees in making more informed healthcare decisions?

2. According to DeVries, studies have shown that acupuncture can help treat ailments that commonly affect employees' performance. What ailments does DeVries mention?

3. What are the three converging issues that are driving Americans' interest in alternative medicines and treatments, in DeVries's view?

The popular strategy for controlling health care costs is to shift a greater share of the cost burden to the shoulders of employees through consumer-driven plan designs. Critics of this strategy say that consumer-driven plans may help reduce immediate damage to an employer's bottom line, but they do nothing to alter the fundamental problems that lead to high healthcare costs, such as poor employee health habits and excessive use of costly health services. Indeed, many argue that these plans unfairly burden low- and moderate-income employees, forcing them to forego preventive care or routine doctor visits because of high out-of-pocket costs. A 2005 survey by the Employee Benefit Research Institute substantiates these concerns. The survey found that one-third of the surveyed individuals in consumer-driven and other high-deductible plans reported skipping or delaying medical care because of costs, as compared to 17% of individuals in comprehensive health plans.

Implementing plans that discourage employees from using preventive care, getting routine checkups or catching a potentially serious illness in its early stages is not a promising strategy for containing health costs. Research shows most health cost increases aren't driven by employee use of routine or preventive care but by chronic conditions, unexpected hospitalizations, expensive medical procedures and prolonged medical treatment.

Fortunately, many employers now are recognizing that the best way to make a significant cost impact is to incorporate a broader range of cost-containment solutions, including employee empowerment strategies. According to a 2006 Deloitte & Touche survey, 38% of employers—as compared to 21% in 2003—had implemented strategies that encourage employees to become better health care consumers and to participate in wellness and disease management programs.

In addition to these empowerment programs, a growing number of employers are adding another prong to their cost-containment strategy—health coverage for complementary and alternative medicine.

Complementary and Alternative Medicine Coverage

Clinical evidence proves that alternative therapies help control medical costs through the phenomenon of *substitution*. Employees migrate to alternative health care when traditional medical care fails them or treatment is not considered acceptable because of cost or potential side effects. Studies show this migration to high-touch, low-cost approaches like chiropractic or massage therapy can significantly reduce an employer's overall medical costs by eliminating or reducing high-tech surgical and pharmacological treatments. In the most compelling study to date [reported in *Archives of Internal Medicine* in October 2001], chiropractic benefits were proven to significantly reduce health care use and costs. The study compared health benefits usage in a group of employees with chiropractic health coverage to a group of employees without chiropractic coverage. In a comparison of the groups, employees with chiropractic coverage experienced 41% fewer hospitalizations due to back pain, 32% fewer back surgeries 37% less use of costly computerized tomography (CT scans) and magnetic resonance imaging (MRI) for back problems, and 23% less use of x-rays. Overall, the cost per episode of treating back pain was 28% lower for employees with chiropractic health plan coverage than for those without coverage.

The study proved access to managed chiropractic care can reduce key cost factors that drive up employer health costs in traditional care settings. With back pain and musculoskeletal disorders costing employers $61 billion per year in lost production time alone, the addition of a chiropratic benefit is something to consider.

Acupuncture and Massage Therapy

Chiropratic care is not the only complementary health therapy that has demonstrated proven clinical success. Research trials and rigorous studies conducted by the National Center for Complementary and Alternative Medicine (NCCAM), in collaboration with the national Centers for Disease Control and Prevention, are proving them is validity in claims about the benefits of many therapies. Most recently, for example, a landmark study demonstrated acupuncture not only provides pain relief but also improves function for people suffering with osteoarthritis of the knee. More than 20 million Americans suffer from osteoarthritis. Other studies showed acupuncture is effective at treating various ailments that impact employees, including chronic headache, menstrual cramps, tennis elbow, fibromyalgia, myofacial pain, lower back pain, carpal tunnel syndrome and asthma.

Several important studies provided clinical evidence that massage therapy is effective in reducing pain and fatigue. As a

Prevention Is the Key to Lowering Costs

With the alternative health sector surging, giant insurers are starting to notice the fact that holistic treatments are cheaper than surgery, a lifetime of prescription refills or Western-style occupational therapy. As a result of personal experience and about 20 years in the insurance business, Steve Gorman, founder of Alternative Health Insurance Services, which helps clients find group insurance plans that cover holistic medicine, believes that alternative therapies are cost effective. "If you can prevent somebody from getting a major illness, even if it costs a little more on the front end . . . that would save tons and tons of money, rather than waiting until someone has a disease and then treating it."

Emily Dulcan, "Naturopathy, Bodywork, Acupuncture . . . Claim Accepted!" Whole Life Times, February 2007. http://wholelifetimes.com.

result of such studies, about 13% of Fortune 200 companies offer massage therapy as part of their employee benefit programs.

As organizations like NCCAM continue to fund a greater number of clinical trials with successful outcomes, use of complementary and alternative medicine is expected to increase.

Reducing Stress-Related Employee Absenteeism and Turnover

Health care costs are 50% higher for workers who report high levels of stress, according to the *Journal of Occupational and Environmental Health*. According to studies by the Bureau of National Affairs, a publisher of legal and regulatory news that affects business and government, 40% of job turnover is related to stress. Stress is so prevalent in the workplace today, and so debilitating, that many employers now allow employees to file workers' compensation claims for emotional disorders and disabilities caused by stress.

Workplace stress costs employers more than $300 billion a year—or $7,500 per employee—through stress-related compensation claims, reduced productivity, absenteeism, health insurance costs, direct medical expenses and employee turnover, according to the National Institute for Occupational Safety and Health.

Enlightened companies are turning to stress management classes and complementary health treatments, such as yoga and massage, to help employees cope. Both massage and yoga are proven methods of triggering physical, emotional and mental changes that can significantly decrease stress, lower absenteeism and enhance productivity. For example, the Touch Research Institute at the University of Miami discovered that a basic 15-minute chair massage provided twice weekly results in decreased job stress and a significant increase in productivity. In addition, anecdotal evidence from large employers about the positive effects of massage has facilitated employer acceptance of this service as a therapy. According to the Society of Human Resource Management, 18% of large employers offer massage therapy as an employee benefit.

Demand for Nontraditional Health Care Options

More and more Americans are turning to nontraditional medical care. They are taking $27 billion per year out of their own pockets for chiropractic, acupuncture, massage and other complementary and alternative health services. The actual number of adult Americans using at least one alternative or complementary treatment is estimated at anywhere from 48% to 62%. Health care experts say this rate will continue to increase rapidly over the next few decades, thanks to the convergence of a number of key issue, including:

- *Increasing Concerns About Mainstream Medicine.*
  Americans' concerns about mainstream medicine
  stem from factors such as difficulty in appointment scheduling, misdiagnosis and medical errors,
  unsatisfactory treatments and the rush to prescribe
  prescription drugs.

- *Increasing Exposure to Alternative Therapies.* Over
  the last several decades, rising immigration rates
  were accompanied by the growth of Eastern medicine practices. This mushrooming of new options
  and a subsequent cross-pollination of medical
  ideas and treatments facilitated the acceptance of
  alternative therapies in mainstream America.

- *Baby Boomer Demand for Novel Approaches.* Baby
  boomers have been bucking the system for the last
  five decades, and they continue to be pioneers
  even into their sunset years. Many are taking their
  health issues into their own hands. In their quest
  for eternal youth, they seek answers through nontraditional practitioners who provide them with a
  more holistic view of health issues by addressing
  emotional, spiritual and environmental factors that
  can impact their physical health.

All in all, this growing national interest in complementary
and alternative medicine therapies provides an opportunity
for employers to rethink the way they approach health benefits and offer less costly substitutes to expensive traditional
therapies.

Benefit Coverage Mandates

Over the past decade, the trend toward alternative care has
been carefully watched by the health care and insurance in-
dustries, as well as state regulators. To ensure access for more

Americans, some states are mandating that insurers cover some form of alternative services. Today more than 40 states require coverage for chiropractic care, while eight require coverage for some form of alternative medicine (acupuncture, naturopathy, massage therapy, etc.). With these mandates expected to further expand, and with the growth of specialty insurers who sell a broad range of complementary and alternative coverage, traditional insults are expanding their complementary care offerings to make purchasing easier for employers.

A plan generally costs 1–2% of an employer's total health care premium. In return, the employer gains recruitment and retention advantages, as well as possible reduced health care costs and absenteeism.

Employers can purchase complementary health plans from traditional insurers in some states, but in areas where coverage is not available or is limited in its scope, the best option is to purchase it directly from a specialty benefits company. Such companies offer the broadest range of coverage and often provide additional health services, such as wellness plans, weight management and smoking cessation.

Complementary and alternative medicine insurance as part of a health care cost-containment strategy is a potential way to lower medical costs, reduce absenteeism and presenteeism, reduce employee turnover and make a benefits package more attractive to prospective employees.

Periodical Bibliography

The following articles have been selected to supplement the diverse views presented in this chapter.

Mark B. Abelson and Lisa Lines	"Why Patients Are Going Back to Nature," *Review of Ophthalmology*, April 2006.
David Baines	"Hard to Swallow," *Canadian Business*, March 27, 2006.
Andrea H. Brockman	"The Great Leap Forward in Marketing Alternative Health: Why Alternative Health Practitioners Should Do More to Educate the Public," *Townsend Letter for Doctors and Patients*, February 1, 2005.
Robert Davis	"Alternative vs. Conventional Medicine," *WebMD Commentary*, December 13, 2005. www.webmd.com.
Economist	"The Wellness Boom," January 4, 2007.
Jerome Groopman	"No Alternative," *Wall Street Journal*, August 7, 2006.
David E. Gumpert	"Old-Time Sales Tricks on the Net: Should a Popular Alternative-Doctor's Web Site Be Allowed to Blur the Lines between Business and Medicine?" *Business Week Online*, May 23, 2007.
Yael Kohen	"Run the New Age Gauntlet," *New York*, January 22, 2007.
Mary Mihaly	"Mind/Body Magazines Evolve," *Writer*, June 2006.
Catherine Price	"Saying Ah to Acupuncture," *Health*, April 2007.
William Triplett	"Dietary Supplements," *CQ Researcher*, September 3, 2004.

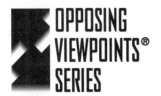

CHAPTER 3

Can Alternative and Conventional Medicine Work Together?

Chapter Preface

In a 2005 edition of *Consumer Reports*, the polling and review magazine reported that while more people were experimenting with complementary and alternative medicine (CAM) than in previous years, not all were in agreement that CAM was effective in treating ailments. Some survey participants acknowledged that CAM made them feel "much better" or helped out "somewhat" in treating health conditions; the majority reported that conventional therapies were more effective. However, two forms of CAM did win praise as being more effective than conventional treatments or drugs. Those polled testified that both chiropractic therapy and deep-tissue massage were ideal for reducing back, neck, and musculoskeletal pains.

From the results, *Consumer Reports* concluded that "most alternatives may make more sense as an adjunct to conventional care than as a primary cure." That is, alternative treatments and herbal medicines may have some power in reducing stress, soothing pain, and maintaining overall health. Thus, they may be excellent resources for preventative care, leaving users less prone to pain and bringing them a new framework for pursuing a healthier lifestyle. Furthermore, the cooperation between conventional and alternative medicine is highlighted in medical institutions through their recent emphasis on integrative medicine, a health philosophy that seeks to take advantage of the benefits of both forms of treatment.

Those who champion integrative medicine claim that it is necessary not merely for its potential medical value but also because doctors need to become familiar with the alternative therapies that their patients are using, whether prescribed or not. Peter A. Clark, writing in the *Journal of Public Health Policy*, stipulates that in order for patients to make informed decisions about health care options, their doctors "should be educating themselves about these alternative therapies, helping patients seek similar reliable information about the safety and effectiveness of these treatments." He makes this assertion because, as he writes, "Alternative medicine is a reality that can no longer be ignored by academia [and] the medical establishment."

In the following chapter, various authors debate whether conventional and alternative medicines can coexist in the modern healthcare field. Some examine practical and methodological disparities that suggest that integrative medicine might be more a convenient term rather than an accurate description of a unified vision of health care. Others follow Clark's prediction that the inevitability of expanded CAM use will compel most physicians to incorporate at least an understanding of alternative treatments into their own practices.

"When frightened or concerned about their health, most people turn to their main source of strength."

Spirituality Should Be Part of Conventional Medical Treatment

Barbara Anan Kogan

Barbara Anan Kogan is a doctor of optometry who writes on health topics for various periodicals. In the following viewpoint, Kogan cites several medical studies that have shown a link between patients' spirituality and their ability to overcome illness. Relying on this connection, Kogan asserts that physicians are looking for ways to address patients' spiritual needs in healthcare settings. The National Center for Complementary and Alternative Medicine, for example, is researching the subject to find methods of using the healing power of spirituality in routine doctor visits as well as in more serious healthcare situations.

As you read, consider the following questions:

1. What were the findings of the Duke University research cited by Kogan?

Barbara Anan Kogan, "Prescription: God—Does What You Believe Affect How Fast You Heal?" *Vibrant Life*, May–June 2006, pp. 13–15. Copyright © 2006 Vibrant Life. Reproduced by permission.

2. As Kogan relates, what were the results of research done in Roseto, PA, between the 1940s and the 1970s?

3. According to the 1998 Harvard survey, cited by Kogan, what percent of Americans reported that prayer was "very helpful" in addressing medical issues? What percent reported that they discussed this with their physicians?

Is spirituality good for your health? The question hangs in the auditorium air as Stephen E. Straus, M.D., director of the National Center for Complementary and Alternative Medicine (NCCAM), looks out over the Christian clergy and local seminary students assembled at the National Institutes of Health (NIH) campus hospital in Bethesda, Maryland. "Does spirituality have a medicinal value alternative to normative procedures?" he continues. "Can we live longer and get better more quickly?"

Harvard University's Anne Harrington, Ph.D., distinguished lecturer for the NCCAM, takes her place behind the podium and begins her response to those questions by pointing to a chart indicating prayer as the number one practice among more than 31,000 adults the center surveyed. Forty-three percent of those polled said that they prayed for their own health, and 24 percent prayed for others as well.

The results of that survey led to federal funding of five NIH studies on prayer, spirituality, and healing. Researchers knew that patients prayed. They wanted to know how and why that simple practice enhanced their health.

Finding Time for Spirituality in the Exam Room

Christian spirituality—as defined by the studies—is the belief an individual has in one God. While 67 percent of doctors surveyed professed a belief in God and 95 percent felt that a patient's spiritual outlook was important to handling health difficulties, less than 20 percent of all patient visits included spiritual factors.

Practitioners felt that lack of time was an important barrier to addressing those elements in their patients' diagnoses. However, a majority stated that proper training in how to manage such issues could overcome those barriers and improve their ability to more fully respond to a patient's spiritual requirements.

To help bridge the gap between patient and health-care provider, the NCCAM defines prayer as "an active process of appealing to a higher spiritual power, specifically for health reasons," and includes individual or group prayer on behalf of one's self or others. The term *spirituality* is broader, defined as "an individual's sense of purpose and meaning in life beyond material values, including religion."

At Johns Hopkins University's Department of Managed Care in Baltimore, Maryland, clinicians measured the spiritual pulse of patients in order to identify perceived barriers to integrating spirituality into their care. They discovered that 90 percent of adults believe in God, 82 percent pray weekly, and a majority want their physicians to address spirituality during a health-care visit.

Dr. Harrington cites that, within the past five years, 70 medical schools have begun offering courses in spirituality and health. With proper post-doctoral medical education training, physicians are learning to gather not only a patient's medical and family health history during an examination, but their spiritual history as well.

The Health Benefits of Religion

Studies have shown that attending church is good for the immune system and allows changes in brain chemicals that "kick-start" many health practices. Increasing scientific research also suggests that not only are religion and spirituality connected

The Danger of Putting Second Things First

The resurgence in interest regarding spiritual matters raises questions about the provision of "spirituality" by healthcare professionals. Medicine's traditional focus on the physical dimensions of health and healing is increasingly being extended to encompass patients' emotional, relational, and spiritual concerns as well. As a result, the door has been opened for discussions between physicians and patients which would not have been possible a few years ago. Although this shift presents Christian physicians with a great opportunity to share their faith, a real danger exists in that patients might become open to matters of faith because they believe it may offer health benefits. This would be, to paraphrase [Christian scholar and author] C. S. Lewis, putting second things first.

Dónal P. O'Mathúna,
"Spirituality & Alternative Medicine in the New Millennium,"
Center for Bioethics & Human Dignity,
April 12, 2001. www.cbhd.org.

directly to mental and physical health, but they also can play a powerful role in the medical treatment of patients with severe chronic illnesses.

Warming to her subject, Dr. Harrington goes on to explain that "Presently, we're dealing with spirituality on a cultural level. Medicine will be better off when we start dealing with spirituality on an ethical level." She adds that patients' immune systems are crying out for spirituality. But doctors can't hear spirituality on their stethoscopes, and therefore, many don't consider it to be medically curative. Harrington declares that an ethical and moral agenda—instead of a purely scientific agenda—should be adhered to by health-care providers.

NCCAM's future studies will also evaluate the curative effects of contemplation, meditation, and faith.

Making the Connection

When frightened or concerned about their health, most people turn to their main source of strength. They don't wait until scientific research creates a framework built on what other people believe. Harrington cites the Seventh-day Adventist Church as being known for the health benefits associated with a vegetarian diet and a strong sense of community—faith elements not always shared by other religions.

North Carolina's Duke University researchers found that when organized religious activities were included in a patient's care, his or her acute-care hospitalization stay was shorter. The robust and persistent effects of religiousness and/or spirituality in long-term health care were well documented as particularly beneficial among African-Americans and women over 50.

Children represent another area of consideration. With the rapidly increasing use of complementary therapies, North Carolina's Wake Forest University School of Medicine researchers also discovered an improved effectiveness in clinical practice and enriched, deepened pediatric patient response during clinical care. The cases, reported in a clinical pediatric journal, supported the use of spirituality-based roleplaying and personal reflection in complementary medicine.

Evidence of the Healing Benefits of Faith

The interest in the possibility that religious and spiritual activity may confer health benefits is increasing. A Columbia-Presbyterian Medical Center director of behavioral medicine feels it's important to conduct clinical trials in order to provide the scientific basis that will allow physicians to make recommendations such as "attend religious services" along with their regular medical treatment.

Dr. Harrington provides a poignant example correlating increased longevity with church attendance within an almost entirely Italian-American tightly knit community in Roseto, Pennsylvania. In the years following World War II, the members of this community boasted the lowest heart-disease rates in the entire United States. An earlier eight-year study found the average life span was 83.

Cardiac mortality in Roseto hovered near zero in men 55 to 64, half the national average in spite of high levels of obesity and other lifestyle risk factors. This led researchers to write about the role of faith and belief in stimulating the ability to heal. The community's spiritual integrity included faith that God could see them through any surgery. Twenty years after the initial Roseto coronary artery disease study, the same spiritual philosophy was being confirmed in other studies.

Americanization and Mortality

However, after 30 years had passed Roseto residents' values and goals were becoming more in line with the more materialistic views held by the residents of nearby Bangor. The death rate from myocardial infarctions (heart attacks) increased to equal that of their less spiritually inclined neighbors. A 50-year Roseto-Bangor comparison completed by nearby Bethlehem, Pennsylvania's Lehigh University, found that the mortality rate increase experienced by the Rosetans was owing to a larger number of younger men and elderly women in the community. The "Americanization" of Roseto, with its reduced solidarity and church attendance, created the matched mortality between these two originally diverse communities.

Texas researchers, in reviewing a national health interview survey on multiple causes of death and its relationship with religious attendance, found that people who never attended church had a 1.87 times higher risk of death than those who attended more than once a week. Nonattendance increased the likelihood of being unhealthy, having a reduced life expectancy of seven years when compared with churchgoers, and dying. Five years after their published study, additional researchers were confirming that religious involvement is linked to mortality risks. The evidence was strongest for *public* religious activity and the weakest for *private* religious activity.

Therapeutic Benefits of Prayer

A San Francisco intercessory prayer (IP) group focused on 192 hospitalized Christian coronary care individuals and compared the results with 201 individuals in a control group without IP. During the 10-month study, members of the IP group experienced a significantly lower severity during their hospitalization; while those in the control group required ventilatory assistance, antibiotics, and diuretic medication more frequently. The collected data suggests that prayer to a Christian God—one of the oldest forms of therapy—produces definite therapeutic benefits. The study also acknowledges that little attention is being devoted to these benefits in modern medical literature.

Harvard Medical School researchers, knowing that prayer is common in the U.S., conducted a national survey of 2,055 individuals in 1998 to determine prayer's prevalence and patterns. They discovered that 35 percent of those surveyed prayed for health concerns, 75 percent went to God concerning their overall wellness, and 22 percent petitioned for specific concerns. While 69 percent found prayer "very helpful," only 11 percent discussed this with their physician.

The Answer Is Yes

Dr. Harrington concludes her remarks at the NIH campus hospital auditorium by saying that multisite national researchers have found that patients experience significant improvement in disease-fighting antibodies after participating in a mindful meditation program. Spirituality and emotional well-being also allowed for alterations in brain structure and immune system functioning. NCCAM-supported researchers report that there is a small but growing body of literature linking faith in God with enhanced health and healing.

Is spirituality good for your health? In study after study, science is uncovering irrefutable evidence to support what people of faith have known for a long, long time.

"Healthcare practitioners simply have no right to influence directly and deliberately the spiritual aspects of patients' lives."

Spirituality Should Not Be Part of Conventional Medical Treatment

Timothy N. Gorski

In the following viewpoint, gynecologist Timothy N. Gorski argues that religion and healthcare need to remain separated. It would be impossible, Gorski states, for physicians to be able to address the varying spiritual needs of their patients. Furthermore, if physicians began incorporating religion into their practices, Gorski warns, they might offend certain believers or nonbelievers and erode the delicate trust between patients and doctors. Indeed, Gorski asserts that patients expect that their right to find their own spiritual counsel will not be subverted by sermonizing doctors. Gorski is also a member of the board of directors of the National Council Against Health Fraud.

Timothy N. Gorski, "Should Religion and Spiritual Concerns Be More Influential in American Healthcare? No," *Priorities*, vol. 12, no. 1, March 1, 2000. Copyright © 1997–2003 American Council on Science and Health. Reproduced with permission of American Council on Science and Health (ACSH). For more information on ACSH visit www.acsh.org.

As you read, consider the following questions:

1. Why does Gorski believe it is unethical for physicians to counsel patients in spiritual matters?
2. What is humanism, as Gorski describes it, and how would incorporating religion into healthcare violate its principles?
3. How would broaching the topic of religion in healthcare add to the numerous "misunderstandings" that undermine the physician-patient relationship, in Gorski's view?

Religious and spiritual concerns have traditionally been in the background in American healthcare, which has relied largely on medical science for guidance. But the medical subordination of such concerns has never given health professionals or healthcare administrators in the United States license to belittle or ignore religious beliefs and practices, which are integral to many persons' sense of well-being. More to the point, it has never meant that patients could not turn to religious practices, or to clerics, for comfort as adjuncts to medical care. Importantly, it has facilitated health professionals' maintaining detachment from patients' religious and private spiritual matters.

This is as it should be, in light of how subjective religious opinions are, how deep-rooted they can be, and their extraordinary diversity in the U.S. If religious and spiritual concerns became more influential in medicine, effective, ethical, compassionate healthcare would suffer. Incorporating religion with medicine would be inconsistent with major ideals of the medical profession:

Remaining Objective

Objectivity A substantial increase in religion's influence on healthcare would result in a decrease in objectivity and impartiality among medical professionals.

Religious Nonpartisanship How can healthcare practitioners actively support their patients' diverse religious beliefs and practices without hypocrisy; without offending patients who do not subscribe to certain of such beliefs; and without offending atheists, agnostics, and religious nonaffiliates, who together constitute a significant proportion of the American population?

In no interfaith, nondenominational, or multicultural healthcare setting can a medical professional exhibit an appeal to Allah without diminishing non-Islamic mainstream religious principles. It is likewise impossible to pray conspicuously to the Virgin Mary or to Roman Catholic saints without encroaching on Protestant beliefs. Many Christians regard even spiritual practices that are neo-Christian, nondenominational, and/or eclectic—particularly those associated with the New Age movement—as harmful, if not devil-inspired. Allegiance to ecclesiastic principles has led to calls for boycotts against Disney and even the U.S. military. Unless American healthcare becomes balkanized on the basis of religious creeds, a substantial increase in religion's influence on medicine would lead to hypocrisy, factionalism, and partisanship within hospitals and clinics.

Those who doubt that increasing religion's influence in healthcare would be divisive can easily rid themselves of such doubt, by becoming informed of recent events in which the intersection of religion and medicine has been crucial—for example, the firing of a physician based on his having submitted a letter to a local newspaper editor that conveyed views his employer described as contrary to fundamental Roman Catholic teachings; the scuttling of hospital-merger plans because of religious orders' steadfast demands concerning what medical services are ecclesiastically acceptable; and clashes over "assisted reproduction," abortion, euthanasia, and other issues on which there is no universal religious consensus. Indeed, the prospect of the spiritualizing of healthcare is appealing only to the extent that one associates such expressions as "religion" and "spirituality" with one's subjective religious and spiritual beliefs.

Respecting Patients' Interests

Nonmaleficence and beneficence Health professionals have a dual responsibility to their patients: to "do no harm" (nonmaleficence) and to act according to the best interests of each patient (beneficence). Both whether religion can improve health and what risks religion may entail are far from determined. Incorporating religion with medicine raises serious questions of medical ethics.

For example, although it appears that churchgoers tend to be healthier and more long-lived than nonchurchgoers, even incontrovertible proof that churchgoers are healthier and more long-lived would hardly constitute a sound basis for the contention that churchgoing per se is responsible for these advantages. The association apparently does not depend on what church is attended. Thus, social connectedness may be at least partly responsible for it. And healthier segments of the American population—e.g., the married, the occupationally satisfied, and the prominent—may tend to be more socially connected. Moreover, perhaps individuals who are healthy and socially well connected are more disposed to churchgoing than are unhealthy, poorly socially connected persons. Therefore, churchgoers may attend religious services partly because they are relatively healthy and partly because they are well connected socially. On the other hand, many of the reasons religiously nonobservant persons have for this nonobservance—for example, familial religious discord—may be such that churchgoing would be unhealthful for them.

Until such questions of causality and contraindications are answered scientifically—if they can be—it is dangerous and ethically unacceptable for healthcare practitioners to counsel patients on spiritual matters. And it might well be so even if such questions were properly and exhaustively answered. For example, would scientific research establishing that believing in Allah is more therapeutic than is believing in Buddha, Yahweh, Jesus, or the Hindu pantheon constitute adequate grounds for medical professionals' promoting Islam to patients over religions associated with the other alleged divine spirits? Furthermore, would scientifically establishing that undergoing a crisis of religious doubt carries serious health risks make it appropriate to deal with such doubt as pathologic and medically remediable? And if it were appropriate, could medical professionals credibly claim an objective understanding of what is best for patients concerning religion?

Patients' autonomy Increasing religion's influence in healthcare would diminish the autonomy of patients. It is incumbent on physicians to know the health advantages and health risks to individual patients of each of numerous validated interventions, and to be prepared to convey such information intelligibly to patients so that the patients can make informed decisions. In matters of religion, however, a hands-off policy should continue to prevail among health professionals, except when the potential health consequences of particular religious behaviors are clear-cut and adverse to the patient—for example, a patient's refusal of a blood transfusion without which he or she would die, or parents' rejection of critical medical care for their underage children.

When the prospective health consequences of particular religious behaviors are not clear-cut, and when they are not adverse to the patient, the religious views and spiritual suggestions of medical professionals are extraneous. Indeed, expressions of such opinions may be unwelcome and, even if they are welcome initially, may introduce coercion into the physician-patient relationship. It is out of a respect for patients' autonomy that the rule of nonjudgmental noninterference has been established for such eventualities as certain nonreligious cultural practices, unusual sex acts, childbearing in various hazardous circumstances (e.g., of the patient's making), and even, to some degree, "recreational drug use." It is ironic that in such cases medical professionals respect individuals' lifestyle choices, for good or ill, as an ethical obligation, while it is seriously and widely proposed that such professionals should urge their patients to pray, attend religious services, and embrace various supernatural beliefs. Aren't religion and spirituality at least as intimate as sexuality, the instinct to reproduce, and nonreligious cultural aspects of personality?

Keeping the Physician-Patient Relationship Intact

Humanism Biomedicine is rooted both in science and in humanism—a philosophy that promotes, for example, not only consideration for the sick and understanding and tolerance of religious beliefs and practices in general, but also acceptance of the rights of conscience of nonreligious persons. Consistency with this long-standing aspect of modern medicine requires that healthcare professionals distance themselves from any purely religious issues that may arise in the context of their duties; it certainly demands that such professionals forbear from promoting and/or challenging religious beliefs, whatever their patients may want in the way of medico-spiritual counseling.

It is very likely that an expansion of the role of religion in healthcare would not humanize medical care but rather would erode, perhaps even devastate, the physician-patient relationship, which has always been the cornerstone of compassionate medical care. A 1999 edition of the Texan paper the *Arlington Morning News* quoted a hometown girl who had recently graduated high school: "I want to be a pediatric surgeon because I really love little kids, and if you work on little kids and they die, then you at least know they will go to heaven since they haven't had time to do anything wrong in their life." The

sentiments behind this statement were undoubtedly inno-
cent—but would such an expression comfort parents with a
desperately ill child being prepped for surgery? And suppose
the parents' afterlife-related beliefs differ markedly from those
that the surgeon's statements suggest.

There are many other risks—subtler than those of diminishing patients' autonomy and privacy—inherent in the en-
croachment of religion on medicine. For example, how would
the role of clergy change? How would relationships change in
interfaith households and among friends of different theolo-
gies? The effects would be unpredictable and, especially in
cases of grave illness, could be perilous. If healthcare professionals—who themselves have disparate religious, antireli-
gious, and secular philosophies—were constrained to incorporate religion and spirituality in their practices, certainly they
would do so differently, and with scarce scientific grounds for
such disparities. Healthcare practitioners simply have no right
to influence directly and deliberately the spiritual aspects of
patients' lives.

In healthcare there are numerous occasions for misunderstandings that can undermine the often fragile physician-
patient relationship. A physician's mispronouncing a patient's
name, addressing a patient by the wrong name, or momen-
tarily forgetting what a patient has just said, for example, can
alone put a dent in their relationship. Physicians' spiritually
pontificating, sermonizing, or even just neutrally broaching
specific religious concepts can only make matters worse. For
instance, how might a patient—particularly a religious non-
Christian patient—react if a physician asked him or her: "Have
you accepted Jesus Christ as your personal savior?"

Traditionally, recourse to religion or to spiritual practices
has figured in biomedical settings in developed countries only
in cases of grave, intractable, or incurable illness. But many
formerly grave, intractable, or incurable diseases are very
treatable; and it is because those ostensible explanations and

remedies that were religious did not satisfy medical professionals that there has been progress against formerly untreatable diseases.

By distancing itself somewhat from religion and spiritual concerns, American healthcare avoids stepping on spiritual and other toes. Incorporating religion with medicine would ultimately please no one. Unions of religious and governmental bodies have long tended to be calamitous. There is no good reason to believe that expanding American healthcare's religious or spiritual features would have different results.

> *"A common set of methods and standards for generating and interpreting evidence is necessary if health care providers are to make informed decisions about the use of both conventional treatments and CAM."*

Alternative Medicine Should Submit to Conventional Testing Standards

The National Academies

In this viewpoint, the Institute of Medicine of the National Academies states that the same research principles and standards for testing a treatment's effectiveness should apply to both conventional medicine and complementary and alternative medicine (CAM). Researchers argue that with the increasing popularity of remedies such as dietary supplements, acupuncture, and naturopathy, there is a need for proper clinical testing of these alternative treatments to ensure the quality of the product and the safety of the patient. The Institute of Medicine is a private, nonprofit organization that offers health policy advice. The Na-

tional Academies brings together committees of experts in all areas of science and technology to address critical national issues and to give advice to the federal government and the public.

As you read, consider the following questions:

1. How many of adults reported having pursued some form of CAM treatments?
2. What criteria did the study use to determine which CAM therapies to prioritize for study?
3. What are among the most widely used forms of CAM?

Stating that health care should strive to be both comprehensive and evidence-based, a new report from the Institute of Medicine of the National Academies calls for conventional medical treatments and complementary and alternative treatments to be held to the same standards for demonstrating clinical effectiveness. The same general research principles should be followed in evaluating both types of treatments, although innovative methods to test some therapies may have to be devised, said the committee that wrote the report.

The committee noted in particular the escalating popularity of dietary supplements as well as the lack of consistency and quality in these products, which are an important component of several complementary and alternative approaches. Product inconsistency hinders health professionals' abilities to guide patients on the use of supplements and researchers' ability to study them. The report calls on Congress to work with stakeholders to amend the regulation of supplements to improve quality control and consumer protections and to create incentives for research on the efficacy of these products.

"Ideally, health care should be comprehensive, grounded in the best available scientific evidence, and centered on patients' needs and preferences," said committee chair Stuart Bondurant, interim executive vice president for health sciences and executive dean, Georgetown University Medical Center,

Washington, D.C. "Health professionals and patients should have sufficient information about safety and efficacy to take advantage of all useful therapies, both conventional and complementary and alternative. To that end, we believe that the same research principles and standards for showing effectiveness should apply to both conventional and complementary and alternative treatments. And because evidence is a key element of prudent decision-making, we need to change the current regulation of dietary supplements in this country to encourage more studies of these widely used products and to ensure their quality," he said.

Written to assist the National Institutes of Health in developing research methods and setting priorities for evaluating products and approaches within complementary and alternative medicine (CAM), the report also assesses what is known about Americans' reliance on these therapies. Use of CAM is widespread among the U.S. public, with more than one-third of adults reporting that they have pursued some form of these treatments, which include products such as herbal remedies, techniques such as acupuncture, and schools of practice such as naturopathy. Fewer than 40 percent of CAM users have disclosed their use of such therapies to their physicians. More than half of physicians report that they would encourage patients to talk to them about using CAM and would refer them for treatments that fall into that category. However, much is still unknown about how and why people use these therapies in conjunction with or in lieu of conventional therapies.

A common set of methods and standards for generating and interpreting evidence is necessary if health care providers are to make informed decisions about the use of both conventional treatments and CAM. It has been argued that characteristics of CAM therapies—such as customization of treatments, variations in how practitioners perform treatments, or the holistic nature of many of these practices—make it difficult to apply traditional clinical studies to them. Randomized controlled trials (RCTs) are the gold standard for providing evidence of efficacy, the committee said, but other study designs can generate useful information on treatments that do not lend themselves to RCTs. Observational studies, case control studies, and studies that specifically measure patients' expectations, emotional states, and other self-healing processes can provide useful data. Some conventional treatments, such as psychotherapy, also have similar characteristics that make them incompatible with RCTs, but they have been successfully evaluated via other methods, the committee noted.

Because many CAM products and approaches have not undergone formal testing and because resources to conduct research are finite, the report outlined several criteria to help determine which CAM therapies to prioritize for study. These same criteria apply equally well to as-yet untested conventional treatments, the committee noted. They include the prevalence and severity of the target health condition; existing evidence that the therapy is effective or may have safety issues; whether there is a plausible biological mechanism by which the therapy might work or the likelihood that research will discover a mechanism; and the likelihood that research will yield unambiguous results. Inability to meet any one of the criteria should not necessarily exclude a therapy from consideration, the report says.

To foster more research on the effectiveness and safety of CAM—as well as on how these therapies compare with one another or with conventional treatments—practitioners need to be trained in research principles and methods. Studies depend on the involvement of those who understand the therapies' characteristics and goals, but CAM training programs focus on preparing students for practice, and few practitioners learn how to conduct research. At the same time, because CAM use is becoming so widespread, all doctors, nurses, and other health care providers should receive education about these treatments during their professional education, the committee urged.

Dietary supplements, such as herbal products and vitamin pills, are among the most widely and increasingly used forms of CAM; use of herbal products jumped 380 percent between 1990 and 1997, for example. The Dietary Supplement Health and Education Act (DSHEA) mandates that supplements be regulated as foods rather than drugs, which means that supplement manufacturers are not required to conduct safety or efficacy tests on their products. Given that manufacturers are not required to conduct testing and are unable to patent many supplements, there is little incentive for supplement makers to invest in research on the effectiveness of these products. Moreover, the general lack of quality control for dietary supplements is problematic because researchers need consistent samples to conduct studies that could further elucidate these products' effectiveness and potential uses, the report says.

The committee also noted that although there are some restrictions on what information and claims can be included on labels, officials at the Federal Trade Commission have described a proliferation of unfounded and exaggerated claims for supplements. This is of concern because many consumers use these products without consulting a health care professional.

To remedy this situation, the report calls on Congress and the appropriate federal agencies to work with industry representatives, researchers, consumers, and other stakeholders to amend DSHEA to implement quality-control standards for each step of the manufacturing process and to enforce more accurate labeling and disclosures and other consumer protections. In addition, the broader regulatory scheme for supplements should be revised to create incentives for privately funded research on the effectiveness of products and brands and on how consumers use these products.

"Any attempt to throw out or discredit CAM [complementary and alternative medicine] on grounds of scientific inadequacy is sure to toss out large portions of conventional medicine alongside."

Conventional Medical Testing Standards Are Flawed

E. Haavi Morreim

In the following viewpoint, E. Haavi Morreim insists that it is unjust to discredit complementary and alternative medicine (CAM) simply because it does not always submit itself to conventional scientific inquiry. As Morreim argues, many conventional drug testing and efficacy measures are flawed and do not guarantee consistent results among patients. In fact, Morreim states that more patients have been harmed by conventionally approved drugs and medical treatments than by alternative therapies. He concludes that if skeptics wish to deny the efficacy of CAM because of scientific inadequacy, then a lot of conventional medicine already in practice will also have to be dis-

E. Haavi Morreim, "A Dose of Our Own Medicine: Alternative Medicine, Conventional Medicine, and the Standards of Science," *Journal of Law, Medicine, and Ethics*, vol. 31, no. 2, Summer 2003, pp. 222–35. Copyright © 2003 by the American Society of Law, Medicine & Ethics. Reproduced by permission of Blackwell Publishers.

missed. Morreim is a professor in the Department of Human Values and Ethics at the University of Tennessee's College of Medicine.

As you read, consider the following questions:

1. What is Morreim's point in discussing the conventional medical practices of artery catheterization, angioplasty, and coronary artery bypass surgery?
2. In Morreim's view, how does funding influence clinical trials of drugs and therapies?
3. In what way is the conventional double-blind drug testing standard inadequate, according to Morreim?

Perhaps the most salient characteristic of conventional medicine is its scientific roots. Particularly at the level of basic science—the anatomy, physiology, biochemistry, and other scientific disciplines that have shown fundamentally what the human body is and how it functions—medicine is profoundly scientific. Moreover, research has led to a variety of stunning successes, such as organ transplants, joint replacements, and the curing or even eradication of infectious diseases that have historically killed many thousands of people. And yet ordinary clinical medicine—the actual practice in which physicians examine individual patients, recommend tests, make diagnoses, and provide treatments—often has rather little resemblance to the tight data and gold-standard rigor of basic science. There are many reasons.

Insufficient Science Is Available

On the most obvious level, there is simply too much to do. The resources of science will probably never be sufficient to permit every phenomenon of human mental and physical function and well-being to be thoroughly studied. And as new technologies are introduced at staggering speed, the task of evaluating their impact and best uses expands the job immeasurably. In addition, no individual physician can possibly keep up with and appropriately incorporate into his practice everything that is known or assimilate the rapid evolution in what becomes known.

However, the ways in which clinical practice stray from science go far beyond this. The medical community has a long history of accepting new technologies, and new uses of existing technologies, with little science to connect theoretical foundations to such practical applications. For instance, pulmonary artery catheterization, widely used for three decades to monitor cardiopulmonary function in critically ill patients, is only now coming under scientific scrutiny as some recent reports suggest it may actually do more harm than good. Similarly, angioplasty to open up clogged arteries in the heart was "performed in hundreds of thousands of patients prior to the first randomized clinical trial demonstrating efficacy in 1992" [according to J. E. Dalen in a 1998 article for *Archives of Internal Medicine*]; likewise, although coronary artery bypass surgery was first performed in 1964, its efficacy was not scientifically evaluated until 1977. And in the case of bypass surgery, most of the patients who receive it are not like the ones in whom it was tested: "only 4 to 13 percent of the patients who now undergo this operation would meet the eligibility criteria for the randomized controlled trials that established its efficacy" [according to A.C. Gellins, N. Rosenberg, and A.J. Moskowitz in a 1998 article for the *New England Journal of Medicine*]. Moreover, this particular surgery is used significantly more in the United States than in Canada and Europe, with no conclusive justification in terms of patients' illness or infirmity.

Methodological Problems

It is also becoming evident that a significant amount of clinical care is based on studies that are methodologically inadequate. For instance, arthroscopic debridement or lavage for osteoarthritis of the knee has been widely practiced, based on theoretical promise and two methodologically limited studies. Recently, a gold-standard randomized, double-blind, placebo-controlled trial showed that this procedure is no better than a sham surgery in which no surgical invasion of the knee took place. Despite the limited evidence supporting the procedure, it has been performed on more than 650,000 people per year.

Similarly, after many years of thinking that hormone replacement therapy (HRT) for postmenopausal women brought a wide variety of benefits—based on observational studies in some cases funded by pharmaceutical companies—only recently has a long-term, double-blind, placebo-controlled trial been completed, suggesting that HRT may, on balance, do more harm than good. The surprising result has prompted many observers to wonder how many more of the well-accepted recommendations issued by conventional medicine are likewise flawed. . . .

The Politics of Funding

In some cases a dearth of science undergirding clinical practices may be the product of nonscientific forces. A research proposal must usually be either commercially or politically attractive if it is to be funded. . . .

A promising, inexpensive approach to treat life-threatening sepsis has struggled to find funding for testing, largely because the major parties have financial stakes elsewhere. In this instance, studies that are promising but small indicate that long-term, low-dose steroids may reduce fatalities from sepsis by as much as 30 percent. However, while the steroids cost around $50, a major pharmaceutical company has recently launched an antisepsis drug costing $7,000 per dose. On one hand, neither that pharmaceutical company nor any other has any financial desire to fund studies for a generic steroid that brings no profit. On the other hand, government agencies like the National Institutes of Health generally fund basic research, not

The Consistency Condition

All data require interpretation and more than one interpretation can usually be made. For example, modern scientific medicine has a preference for interpretations that are consistent with previous theories, "the consistency condition." At times, this works for the benefit of science, but, at other times, particularly in dealing with observations that are truly novel, it may retard the development of science. While much of CAM lies within the current boundaries of science, some is truly novel so may tend to be marginalized or rejected out of hand because of these biases. Also, biased interpretations purporting to be scientific analysis have been used to support the assertion that CAM modalities are not efficacious; while there is not as much scientific evidence that CAM is effective, there is also very little evidence of ineffectiveness.

Robert M. Sade,
"Introduction: Complementary and Alternative Medicine:
Foundations, Ethics, and Law," Journal of Law, Medicine, & Ethics,
vol. 31, no. 2, 2003, pp. 183–190.

clinical drug-testing. Hence, [as T. M. Burton wrote in a 2002 issue of the *Wall Street Journal*] "a Catch-22: Because money is unavailable, only small studies are possible. Because they are small, they are viewed as less than convincing, allowing skepticism to persist—and money to remain unavailable. The drugs that draw the industry's heavy research and promotional money are the branded ones, which are also far more expensive."

Such economic factors are hardly strangers to the conduct of scientific research. Even where basic science is supported by noncommercial resources, much of the science that translates biology into medical drugs, devices, and procedures is the product of commercial enterprise. This is not to say that such research is necessarily tainted or invalid. Drug and device manufacturers, after all, have produced some of medicine's most stunning successes. Rather, it is to say that the direction of the research and the methodology of study are inevitably shaped by the goals of those who sponsor the research. And therapeutic projects that have no sponsors tend to languish. . . .

Slow Incorporation of Science into Practice

Even aside from such scientific potholes, clinical practice often does not reflect the available science. As noted by the Institute of Medicine:

> In the current health care system, scientific knowledge about best care is not applied systematically or expeditiously to clinical practice. An average of about 17 years is required for new knowledge generated by randomized controlled trials to be incorporated into practice, and even then application is highly uneven. . . . The extreme variability in practice in clinical areas in which there is strong scientific evidence and a high degree of expert consensus about best practices indicates that current dissemination efforts fail to reach many clinicians and patients, and that there are insufficient tools and incentives to promote rapid adoption of best practices.

That variability has been widely documented by researchers like John Wennberg, whose Dartmouth Atlas surveying nationwide health care practices indicates that the amount of care provided to patients depends far more on the supply of facilities than on the actual needs of patients. In the federal Medicare program, for instance, "supply-sensitive" services such as specialist consultations, hospitalization, and physician visits have been shown to vary widely, in ways unrelated to patient needs, and with no discernible impact on health outcomes or life expectancy. The discrepancies allegedly generate excess spending up to $40 billion per year. . . .

The Rush of Innovation

In reply to all this it might be argued that such problems are simply happenstance, that medical practice can be improved and made more scientific. To be sure, great efforts are now under way and many of them will improve the quality and scientific basis of health care. However, there will always remain a profound disconnect between medical science and clinical medicine. Science is the study of the general, while clinical medicine is the study of the particular. For a host of reasons, ranging from resource constraints to human complexity to the ethical limits on acceptable research, it will forever be impossible to do medical science in a way that makes ordinary medical care a straightforward matter of applying science to generic patients.

For one thing, over the past few decades "an explosion has occurred in the proliferation and supply of drugs, the availability of technological tests and bedside procedures, and the array of high-tech diagnostic methods and invasive therapeutic maneuvers" [writes A. R. Feinstein in a 1997 issue of *Archives of Internal Medicine*]. The changes are so enormous, pervasive, and rapid that it is essentially impossible for physicians—or anyone else, for that matter—to keep abreast of the developments.

In that vein, some areas at the forefront of medicine change so rapidly that it is difficult to achieve scientifically worthwhile results. By the time enough research subjects are enrolled to provide statistical significance in a clinical trial, physicians' experience and with it their use of the technology have evolved so far that the data are already outdated. This phenomenon was observed in the early use of ECMO (extracorporeal membrane oxygenation) technology, for instance, as well as a host of other cutting-edge interventions.

Inadequacy of the Double-Blind

On a more commonplace level, it must also be understood that the more scientifically pristine a study is, the less it actually applies to ordinary people. Science's gold standard, the randomized, double-blind, controlled trial, is particularly problematic. To rest strictly for the effects of the intervention under investigation, study design must use narrow eligibility criteria. Usually enrollees must suffer exclusively from the particular condition being studied, with a minimum of other diseases and medications, lest research results be confounded by ancillary factors. Once the study is complete, however, it is applied in clinical practice to all those complex patients who would never have been eligible to be test subjects in the study. . . .

An important implication of this misfit between scientific studies' narrowly identified participants and the broad spectrum of people who later receive a given medical intervention is that sometimes even well-researched new drugs and procedures must be quickly withdrawn from the market, as they suddenly produce undesirable results and side-effects that were not seen during the research period. Between September 1997 and September 1998, five drugs approved by the Food and Drug Administration (FDA) were removed from the market because of unexpected side-effects or interactions with other drugs. . . .

Problematic Double Standards

From the foregoing, one can only conclude that the actual clinical practice of medicine cannot realistically, faithfully claim to be the scientific enterprise that is presupposed when CAM [complementary and alternative medicine] modalities are criticized as being "unscientific." Medicine has strong roots in science, and the scientific method has produced many wonderful diagnostic and therapeutic tools. But the actual process of daily clinical care often is, and in many ways must inevitably be, rather far removed from those scientific roots. . . .

The upshot is clear enough. Any attempt to throw out or discredit CAM on grounds of scientific inadequacy is sure to toss out large portions of conventional medicine alongside. To "hold" both to "the same" standards appears to bode far worse for medicine than for CAM.

Hence, one important step toward resolving the tension is to avoid double standards in which CAM modalities are held to a standard of proof that medicine cannot possibly meet. The successes of alternatives cannot be dismissed as mere "anecdotes" and "testimonials," if from conventional providers we accept case reports, case series, observational data, and physicians' statements that "my patients have done well/poorly with this treatment" or "in my clinical experience X has been true." When alternative providers emphasize individualizing care, they should not be called "unscientific" if, at the same time, physicians who also individualize their interventions are approvingly seen to practice the "art" of medicine. A CAM modality should not be singled out as "peddling false hope" if, in a comparable situation, physicians might paint overly optimistic pictures and offer treatments they know will not likely help, on the ground that "we can't take away the patient's hope."

> "Despite the popularity, economic impact and possible benefit of CAM therapies, there is a distinct lack of CAM content across many medical school curricula."

Alternative Medicine Should Be Integrated into Medical School

Philippe Szapary

Dr. Philippe Szapary is an assistant professor of internal medicine at the University of Pennsylvania School of Medicine. In the following viewpoint, Szapary argues that complementary and alternative medicine (CAM) should be integrated into medical school curricula. Szapary bases his claim on the fact that many people are already using CAM, yet a large percentage of doctors and medical students are still not familiar with alternative therapies and medicines

As you read, consider the following questions:

1. What does Szapary say was traditionally assumed to be the reason that people turn to alternative medicine? What did a 1998 survey conclude was a more significant factor in the appeal of alternative medicine?

Philippe Szapary, "Why Teach Complementary and Alternative Medicine to Medical Students?" *www.med.upenn.edu*, May 2007. Reproduced by permission of the author.

2. According to 1998 surveys, what percentage of medical school curricula in the United States included courses in complementary and alternative medicine?

3. What does Szapary say is the first priority in order to successfully develop CAM classes in medical schools?

Complementary and alternative (CAM) medicine refers to those practices explicitly used for the purposes of medical intervention, health promotion, or disease prevention, which are not routinely taught at US medical schools, nor routinely underwritten by third party payers within the existing US health care system. This definition, as proposed by Dr. [David H.] Eisenberg in 1993, becoming rapidly outdated, as medical schools and insurance companies have begun to recognize the importance and value of CAM. The National Center for Complementary and Alternative Medicine (NCCAM) has divided CAM practices into seven major categories: Mind-Body Medicine, Alternative Medical Systems, Lifestyle and Disease Prevention, Biologically-based Therapies, Manipulative and Body-based Systems, Biofield and Bioelectromagnetics.

Trends and Costs

While the definition of CAM may be the subject of some debate, the importance of this movement in modern medicine is not debated. In 1993, a national survey of 1,539 Americans found that 34% used at least one unconventional therapy in the previous year. A follow-up survey in 1997 found that users of CAM services had increased to 42%. Surprisingly, this study found that the number of visits to CAM providers (624 million) exceeded the total number of visits to all primary care providers (386 million) for 1997. Also, the initial survey published in 1993 found that the highest use of CAM services was found in white adults aged 25 to 49 with advanced education and upper income levels. A [2000] estimate of dietary supplement usage conducted jointly by National Public Radio

(NPR), the Kaiser Family Foundation and Harvard's Kennedy School of Government found that race, income and education gap is narrowing as CAM gains more popularity. This survey of 1200 randomly selected adults found that 44% of regular users of dietary supplements were older than 50 years and that 22% were classified as non-white. From an economic perspective, expenditures for CAM professional services were estimated at $21.7 billion in 1997, with $12.2 billion out-of-pocket expenses. Surprisingly, these costs exceeded the total out-of-pocket expenditures for all US hospitalizations.

Reasons for CAM Usage

It was initially believed that patients used CAM therapies because they feel alienated from modern medicine. However, a [1998] national survey of 1035 adults found that disenchantment was less of a predictor of CAM usage, rather patients feel that CAM gives them a sense of empowerment, and it appeals to their holistic philosophy to health, where mind, body and spirit are inextricably linked. This was echoed by Drs. [Ted] Kaptchuk and Eisenberg who wrote that CAM offers patients a "participatory experience of empowerment and authenticity when illness threatens their sense of intactness." Regardless of the reasons for using CAM therapies, it is estimated that 60% of patients still do not discuss CAM therapies with their providers.

Why Physicians Need to Know About CAM

As discussed above, the number of Americans engaged in CAM is increasing and a large proportion of patients do not discuss CAM with their physicians. In teaching the evidence-based practice of medicine, it is important to recognize that some therapies, like acupuncture and gingko biloba have been shown to be effective for selected conditions. Similarly, recent clinical trials suggest that garlic, the fourth best selling botanical in the US, is not as effective in reducing serum cholesterol as initially thought. As patients use CAM therapies with medications, the question of harm is especially important since certain therapies, such as ingestion of ephedra, chaparral, and comfrey, have been reported to be dangerous. Additionally, since an estimated 15 million people use dietary supplements along with prescription medication, there exists the possibility of harmful drug-supplement interactions. Thus it is imperative that all physicians, regardless of their stage in training, be able to help patients interpret claims made by manufacturers of dietary supplements as well as reinforce healthy lifestyle choices. While Healthy People 2010 does not specifically address CAM, it does state that "nutrition education and counseling should be included in all routine health contacts with health professionals."

State of CAM Education

Despite the popularity, economic impact and possible benefit of CAM therapies, there is a distinct lack of CAM content across many medical school curricula. The current status of CAM content in undergraduate medical education (UME), graduate medical education (GME) and continuing medical education (CME) programs are summarized below.

Undergraduate Medical Education (UME)

A growing body of medical knowledge and significant time constraints have made medical school curricula difficult to change. [Since 1990], the Association of American Medical Colleges (AAMC) has urged all US medical schools to update their curriculum in order to keep abreast of the ever changing health care landscape. This medical education reform affords an opportunity to integrate non-traditional topics, such as nutrition, managed care, and CAM into various existing courses and as stand-alone classes. In 1998, the AAMC Report on Medical School Objectives Project refers to the importance of physicians being "sufficiently knowledgeable in both traditional and non-traditional modes of care to provide intelligent guidance to their patients." In 1999, the American Medical Students Association (AMSA) released a statement addressing the need for medical administrators and faculty to "meet the demands of their students by developing and implementing appropriate training in alternative medicines."

In response to these challenges, many medical schools have begun to offer varying amounts of CAM education. One survey of 117 US medical schools in 1998 by [Miriam] Weitzel, found that 75 (64%) offered some form of CAM education, usually as part of an elective. Unfortunately, this descriptive study does not provide details about the structure, organization, and content of curricula and the authors state that there are tremendous "heterogeneity and diversity in content structure and requirements among US medical schools." Also absent from medical school curricula are CAM electives and integrated CAM content across all four years of medical school. The Canadian experience is similar with 12 of the 16 medical schools (75%) offering some CAM education and two Canadian schools offering some practical instruction in specific CAM therapies. Although substantial efforts have begun to introduce medical students to CAM, a significant need exists for a truly integrated curriculum that incorporates CAM concepts across the four years of medical training and is linked to residency education.

Graduate Medical Education (GME)

Less is known about the availability of CAM specific training in US residency programs. To date, GME supervisory review boards, such as the Accreditation Council of Graduate Medical Education (ACGME) and the Residency Review Committee (RRC) have not yet incorporated CAM competencies into the standard medical curriculum for residency programs. For General Internal Medicine (GIM), the RRC does not mention CAM specifically, but it does emphasize the development of

The Attitudes of 266 Medical Students Concerning CAM	Men			Women		
	% Agree	% Neutral	% Disagree	% Agree	% Neutral	% Disagree
Clinical care should integrate the best of conventional and CAM practices.	80.0	12.3	7.7	94.8	4.4	0.8
The results of CAM are in most cases due to a placebo effect.	30.8	33.8	35.4	18.5	29.6	51.9
CAM therapies not tested in a scientific manner should be discouraged.	53.1	17.7	29.2	34.1	27.4	38.5
While a few CAM approaches may have limited health benefits, they have no true impact on treatment of sysmptoms, conditions, and/or diseases.	9.2	16.9	73.9	3.0	7.4	89.6
CAM is a threat to public health.	8.5	10.0	81.5	3.0	7.4	89.6
Health professionals should be able to advise their patients about commonly used CAM methods.	83.8	13.1	3.1	88.9	8.1	3.0
CAM practices should be included in my school's curriculum.	71.5	13.1	15.4	88.1	6.7	5.2
Knowledge about CAM is important to me as a student/future practicing health professional.	81.5	10.0	8.5	94.8	3.7	1.5

TAKEN FROM: Ranjana Chaterji et al., "A Large Sample Survey of First-and Second-Year Medical Students Attitudes toward Complementary and Alternative Medicine in the Curriculum and in Practce," *Alternative Therapies*, vol. 13, no. 1, January/February 2007.

humanistic qualities and skills in patient counseling and preventive medicine. [In one 1998 study, F.B.] Milan and colleagues report a primary care GIM house staff CAM curriculum which consists of three, 2-hour didactic lectures and two half-day sessions with a CAM practitioner. Although the authors did not describe a formal curriculum evaluation, the feedback from the house staff was positive.

The American Academy of Family Practice (AAFP) also publishes core educational guidelines for Family Medicine residents which states that residents should be knowledgeable about the role of vitamins, minerals, antioxidants and spirituality in health and disease. Residents should also be skilled at counseling patients about healthy lifestyles and self-care as well as stress management. More recently, the Society of Teachers of Family Medicine (STFM) published curriculum guidelines specifically addressing CAM which we [the university of Pennsylvania] have adapted. These knowledge, skills, and attitude objectives are the culmination of two years of discussions among this group and can be broadly applied to any primary care residency training program. At the fellowship level, a CAM integrative family medicine fellowship at the University of Arizona exists, but there is no published data describing the experience. The inclusion of CAM into GME is still in its infancy but will likely expand as residents, especially those in the primary care, are faced with advising patients on the safety and efficacy of CAM therapies. What is needed is an innovative CAM elective for all primary care residencies that incorporates didactic, experiential and self-study components to acquaint residents with CAM therapies, help them work with CAM providers and raise important clinical questions for research.

Continuing Medical Education (CME)

In many ways, educating practicing physicians and medical school faculty is a key component to develop a successful CAM curriculum. This is because many physicians, while interested in CAM, lack the knowledge and skills to adequately teach or precept trainees. This point was recognized by the STFM which state that "faculty development must be a first priority" in order to implement a CAM curriculum. Little is known about practicing physicians attitudes on CAM. One [1998] survey of 783 primary care physicians by [Brian] Berman and colleagues indicated that while physicians had little training in CAM, they were generally accepting of CAM and referring patients to CAM providers. Over half of surveyed physicians viewed acupuncture, massage and hypnotherapy as legitimate, and 20% had used chiropractic, hypnotherapy and meditation in the care of their patients. The authors concluded that "when educational opportunities are provided to physicians to assist them with the practice and treatment decisions, the best interests of their patients will be served." At the University of Pennsylvania Health System (UPHS), an unpublished survey of 1500 physicians found that 388 provided some form of CAM therapy to their patients (27% response rate). Although this response rate was low, 45% of those who responded referred patients to CAM therapies.

Computers in Medical Education

There is no doubt that computer technology has forever changed the landscape of medicine. This was recognized early by the AAMC which issued recommendations for the reform of medical education, known as the "General Professional Education of the Physician (GPEP) Report" in 1984. As part of this report, computer technology was encouraged as a vehicle to foster independent learning. Following the GPEP report, the "AAMC published Educating Medical Students: Assessing Change in Medical Education—The Road to Implementation (ACME-TRI)." This report urged medical schools to give medical students a strong grounding in the use of computer technology to manage information, support patient care decisions, select treatments, and develop their abilities as life-long learners. In 1999 the Medical Informatics Advisory Panel of the AAMC outlined some specific educational objectives to help guide medical schools in preparing their graduates for the practice of medicine in the 21st century. The report recognized that medical education is a life-long process that begins in medical school, extends into residency, and continues throughout the years of medical practice. As life-long learners, physicians need to be facile with computers and the internet which allows for private, portable 24-hours/day access to a vast amount of medical information. More importantly, physicians need to be able to retrieve, filter, evaluate and reconcile this massive amount of information.

CAM Content and the Web

While there is no published literature on the quality of CAM information on the Web, the Internet has certainly become a major source of health information for consumers. Unfortunately, the quality of CAM information is very variable and both patients and providers may become confused and frustrated. There is also a distinct lack of free, high quality Web sites designed specifically for physicians to help them navigate the world of CAM in a simple, evidence-based and non-threatening setting. Most CAM Web sites are discipline specific and usually contain a searchable database of published literature. Other good sites are meta-index sites based at Academic centers or the Federal Government and are aimed at providers and sophisticated consumers. At this time [ca. 2000], we did not identify any CAM Education Web sites that provide an interactive platform combining video, audio and evidence-based referenced texts with direct links to a few key databases. Such a site would appeal to all medical "trainees" regardless of their baseline CAM knowledge.

Much Remains to Be Done

In summary, while considerable progress has been made in recognizing the importance of CAM in medical education, much remains to be done. The bounty of information on CAM has yet to be fully integrated within the UME, GME and CME programs in most academic medical centers, despite the recognition that CAM is widely used by patients and that physicians refer patients for CAM therapies and in some instances practice CAM therapies themselves. The explosion of the internet as a forum for both patient and physician health education gives us the unique opportunity to create a high quality Web-based CAM Education Program across the continuum of medical education. Few CAM education Web sites are specifically targeted at health care professionals, and the majority of primary care physicians, who are most likely to impact the success or failure of efforts to integrate CAM, often lack the knowledge and skills necessary to effectively educate patients, residents, and students. Medical schools and Health Systems have not traditionally welcomed CAM, to such an extent that the current definition of CAM defines it, as those therapies NOT taught in medical schools. By developing, implementing, evaluating, and disseminating an innovative model for a Web-based CAM Education Program, we hope this will change.

> *"To my knowledge, there are no formal standards for teaching about CAM [complementary and alternative medicine] in medical schools."*

Alternative Medicine Should Be Evaluated Critically in Medical School

Wallace Sampson

Wallace Sampson is an emeritus professor of medicine at the Stanford University School of Medicine. In the following viewpoint, Sampson states that school medical programs have become too willing to incorporate alternative medicine classes into the curriculum despite the fact that alternative medicine has not been proven effective in treating health complaints. The fact that these courses have been allowed to exist, Sampson argues, is ethically questionable because they do not adhere to the standards of testing used in conventional medical research. Sampson maintains that if students are to be exposed to alternative medicine, then they should be taught to examine these methods critically to determine their efficacy.

Wallace Sampson, "The Need for Educational Reform in Teaching about Alternative Therapies," *Academic Medicine*, vol. 76, no. 3, March 2001, pp. 248–50. Reproduced by permission of the author.

154

As you read, consider the following questions:

1. According to Sampson, what is one way in which practitioners of alternative medicine elevate their treatments while reducing the credibility of conventional medicine?

2. In Sampson's Stanford class, how does he use a magician to question some of the claims of alternative medicine?

3. In Sampson's view, how have medical schools allowed for a double-standard in their teaching practices?

The past 30 years have seen increased interest in CAM [complementary and alternative medicine]. But its level of acceptance is not warranted, as many CAM claims have been convincingly disproved or remain unproved. One reason for CAM's high level of acceptance is the movement's attempt to alter standards for validity. Some CAM advocates propose expanding such standards to include the acceptance of historical traditions, subjectivity, ritual, personal experience, and transcendental experience. Others claim that their systems supply emotional support and cultural meaning to illness and that such support may improve [the] course of specific diseases. Although some advocates accept common standards and participate in Cochvane Collaboration review for evidence, others reject accepted approaches of controlled clinical trials and other testing methods for traditional medicines and therapies as being not appropriate for certain areas of CAM.

Mainstream Acceptance

Even though some CAM concepts represent a sharp deviation from the accepted ways of evaluating medical therapies, an unidentified number of physicians and social scientists in the academic community support them. Indeed, many CAM claims have reached a high level of acceptance despite insufficient scientific support. As a result, government and large foundations generously fund the study of disproved methods and the integration of other methods. Unfortunately, some governmental panels have reached erroneous conclusions, while claiming to have based those conclusions on clinical trial evidence. A case in point is the practice of acupuncture, which was approved for certain uses by a consensus conference of the National Institutes of Health, although the predominance of evidence from the scientific literature demonstrates acupuncture's ineffectiveness except as a placebo or conditioning agent. Another example is the Agency for Health Care Policy and Research's recommendation of manipulation for back pain, even though the evidence for the usefulness of this therapy is largely negative. With inadequate approaches that fail to uphold criteria for validity and plausibility, so-called "evidenced-based" medicine remains fluid and loses its value to help physicians discern what is truly useful.

Other expert students of the field are speaking out with their opinions about CAM's lack of scientific validity. In a [2000] article published after the present [viewpoint] was written, [Paul] Knipschild [of the University of Limburg in Maastricht, Netherlands] reviewed briefly his conclusions after developing and reporting numerous systematic reviews and meta-analyses of "alternative" methods. While opining that although findings are dubious, there is room for more rigorous trials of acupuncture ("Among the better trials some are positive but many others are negative") and effectively dismissing homeopathy ("ridiculous") and whole herb therapies (he reports that the data are inconsistent), he concluded, "I still believe that, in general, alternative treatments do not work." CAM advocates coined the terms "alternative," "complementary," and "integrative" to increase CAM's acceptance. The terms obscure the fact that the methods they describe are, in fact, unproved or disproved. At the same time, advocates use slogans and myths to diminish the authority of biomedicine's scientific tradition. "Doctors do not know anything about nutrition" demeans standard medicine and medical education. "Cut, burn, and poison" demonizes cancer care. The myth

The White House Commission Supports Critical Evaluation in Medical School

CAM taught in the context of conventional medical education should be evidence-based. New educational programs for physicians need to be developed that include the conceptual basis of CAM practices, along with a critical review of the safety and efficacy of CAM practices and products. This information should be incorporated into required courses of medical school curricula and graduate training programs, not relegated to electives, whose content may not be critically evaluated. While many CAM courses are taught from either an advocacy or neutral view, all CAM courses should be taught critically.

White House Commission on Complementary and Alternative Medicine Policy, "Final Report," March 2002. www.whccamp.hhs.gov.

that "only 10–15% of medicine is proved" reduces medicine's credibility and elevates the perceived worth of CAM methods.

CAM in the Curriculum

Because of the concerns stated above and my observation that many courses that had CAM components were being taught either from an advocacy view or from a "neutral" view—in neither case considering content validity—I surveyed U.S. medical schools in 1995–1997 to learn of their approaches to CAM in their curricula. Representatives of all 125 schools surveyed responded, either to the questionnaire or by phone.

The findings of the survey were not encouraging. Of the 56 schools that had some form of relevant course offering, only nine had invited critical lecturers on occasion; their courses were otherwise generally supportive of CAM. Two course directors claimed to present information "neutrally," but did not teach critical methods or invite critical lecturers.

Only four courses either presented a critical orientation or offered critical arguments in a way that significantly investigated advocacy arguments.

Since the time of that survey, courses in medical schools concerning CAM have increased from 38 credit courses to 150 such courses in 70 schools. I suspect, however, that the level of skepticism and investigation of CAM claims has not risen from the level disclosed in the 1995–1997 survey. In fact, my own informal observations in November 2000 of 15 randomly selected courses at various medical schools revealed that none had added critical analysis to the course content.

In 1996 the Office of Alternative Medicine (OAM)—now the National Center for Complementary and Alternative Medicine (NCCAM)—convened a three-day meeting on professional school CAM education in the United States. The meeting reviewed various courses and methods of teaching. All sectarian systems and methods were implicitly accepted as effective. Teaching-method evaluation was not addressed, and concern about validity was mentioned only in one address by a dean of a medical school. Courses on acupuncture and chiropractic were accepted in the same context as other courses. OAM organizers did not invite the directors of critically-oriented courses to speak. I do not believe that NCCAM's approach to professional education shows much improvement from that demonstrated at the 1996 meeting.

The Stanford Course

In the 1970s student-sponsored lecture series at Stanford University School of Medicine featured speakers whose claims for alternative methods conflicted with rational thought and accepted knowledge. In 1979, after faculty indicated their interest in investigating the validity of CAM claims, I was encouraged to develop a course that I still teach in which students learn how to examine claims factually.

The course, Alternative Medicine—A Scientific Perspective, is modeled after two others existing at that time, one at the Loma Linda University School of Dentistry and one at San Francisco State University School of Public Health. The Stanford course operates on the general principle that science proceeds via a series of statements based on accurate observations and subsequent attempts at proof and disproof. Using this approach, claims for unproved methods are considered suspect. Students are taught to think critically about such claims and are introduced to tools for investigating them.

The course is given for two hours per week for nine weeks. The first segments explore sources of human error that contribute to misperceptions and to drawing incorrect conclusions. Guest psychologists discuss primitive modes of thought, perceptual and cognitive errors, cognitive dissonance, memory faults, and belief formation and perseverance—all associated with unproven medical belief systems. A magician demonstrates principles of misperception, misdirection, legerdemain—such as psychic surgery, and ideomotor action—such as dowsing, pendulum diagnosis, and mind reading. These and other sources of misperceived medical experiences form the bases for testimonials and unproved claims.

Other classes explore phenomena that contribute to placebo experience, including counterirritation, suggestion, expectation, consensus, conditioning and reinforcement, the natural history of illness, and regression toward the mean. Then others explore language distortion, myths, propaganda techniques, and cult-like behavior, the last sometimes presented by former cult members. Other subjects include mathematical and statistical approaches to coincidences, and probability problems, including prior probability and Bayes' theorem. The final sessions of the first half of the course concentrate on reading scientific and medical literature, principles of clinical trials, and the analysis of famous errors in science.

Students Become More Discerning

The last half of the course explores specific subjects, such as electromagnetic fields, vitamins and supplements, acupuncture, homeopathy, Laetrile, and other anomalous cancer therapies. Students learn methods for recognizing misinformation in medical literature. In some years, the course includes consideration of the role of dysfunctional and somatiform syndromes in CAM claims. The schedule is flexible, accommodating subjects such as books by Carlos Castaneda, quantum mechanics and consciousness, and the roles of prayer and "touch" therapies. In some years, students make a field trip to a "Whole Life Expo."

Representatives of CAM systems present talks, followed by students' evaluations using methods learned in the first half of the course. (CAM lecturers understand that they cannot report their presentations on their curriculum vitae or in advertisements.) Students are encouraged to examine a specific method or substance of interest to them. Individual students have chosen on-site visits to acupuncture clinics and other offices, where they may receive treatments or merely observe—they then report their experiences to the class. They are encouraged to relate their subjective experiences and to analyze the material objectively, juxtaposing the two descriptions.

By the end of the course, students are expected to be able to gauge the validity of CAM claims, understand those claims' subjective attraction, and appreciate the values of truly complementary methods. These include relaxation, music, massage, art, poetry, body movement, and forms of meditation. These are methods that enhance adjustment, help reduce symptoms, and add a sense of meaning to the experience of illness.

I have outlined the components of this course above in hopes that others will be encouraged to use similar critical approaches when beginning or revising courses dealing with CAM.

Need for Reform

To my knowledge, there are no formal standards for teaching about CAM in medical schools. If a survey similar to mine were done today, it would probably reveal that most CAM information taught in medical schools continues to be ideologically or advocacy-based, or is taught without concern for a therapy's or system's validity. Medical schools have allowed a double-standard system for teaching. At one extreme, the standard allows instruction about CAM as a set of viable systems of knowledge that can be integrated into practice. And even if the course teaches only about CAM therapies—which is more common—it provides little or no critical analysis. The other standard, applied to the usual curriculum subjects, demands both basic scientific validity and clinical evidence-based confirmation.

A consortium of medical schools recently agreed to integrate CAM into their curricula through an evidence-based approach. However, evidence-based analysis of clinical trials is not sufficient to establish validity. Systematic reviews do not incorporate individual reports' errors, inconsistencies, misrepresentations, or subsequent refutations. Nor do they consider plausibility or prior probability based on non-trial data or basic scientific evidence. Such evidence points to the implausibility of "therapeutic touch," homeopathic principles, and manipulative therapy, all of which require extraordinary clinical evidence prior to acceptance.

While I believe that the consortium's approach is one step in the right direction, it is not enough. It is time for all medical schools to make a concerted effort to formally include in their curricula ways to teach students to analyze and critically assess the content validity of CAM claims.

Periodical Bibliography

The following articles have been selected to supplement the diverse views presented in this chapter.

Stephen Barrett — "Some Thoughts about Faith Healing," *Quackwatch.com*, March 3, 2003.

Christine Ann Barry — "The Role of Evidence in Alternative Medicine: Contrasting Biomedical and Anthropological Approaches," *Social Science & Medicine*, June 2006.

Stuart Bondurant and Harold C. Sox — "Mainstream and Alternative Medicine: Converging Paths Require Common Standards," *Annals of Internal Medicine*, January 18, 2005.

Benedict Carey — "Can Prayers Heal? Critics Say Studies Go Past Science's Reach," *New York Times*, October 10, 2004.

Linda L. Isaacs — "Evaluating Anecdotes and Case Reports," *Alternative Therapies*, March–April 2007.

Charles Marwick — "Complementary Medicine Must Prove Its Worth," *British Medical Journal*, January 2005.

Erik Ness — "Faith Healing," *Prevention*, December 2005.

Donal P. O'Mathuna — "Spirituality & Alternative Medicine in the New Millennium," *Center for Bioethics and Human Dignity*, April 12, 2001.

Ajs Rayl — "Integrative Medicine Gains a Mainstream Foothold," *Applied Neurology*, October 1, 2005.

Mark Szostczuk — "Philosophy of Chiropractic and Alternative Healing," *New Life Journal*, July 2006.

Michael Wines — "Between Faith and Medicine: How Clear a Line?" *New York Times*, August 18, 2004.

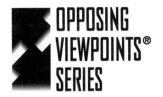

CHAPTER 4

What Should Government Do to Research and and Regulate Alternative Medicine?

Chapter Preface

The U.S. government has maintained, since 1991, that alternative medicine is worth researching and funding. In that year, Congress formed the Office of Alternative Medicine (OAM) within the National Institutes of Health (NIH). Eight years later, the newly inaugurated National Center for Complementary and Alternative Medicine (NCCAM) replaced the OAM and became one of twenty-five official centers within the NIH. In 2000, the NCCAM issued its first strategic plan, a mission statement that lists the goals of the organization over a five-year period (2001–2005). The first strategic plan charted the formation of the organization and showed the NCCAM's intention to fund and follow through on clinical trials relating to alternative medicines and therapies. From trials conducted with NCCAM funding, over 700 scholarly reports were published; a number of these questioned the efficacy of several herbal medicines, while others called for refining research methods.

In 2005, the center initiated its second strategic plan (2005–2009) to expand on the research done in the first five-year term and to launch new inquiries. In its opening paragraphs, the second strategic plan states, "Our aims are very ambitious. NCCAM does not expect to achieve all its objectives in the next 5 years; some will be completed, while others will only have started." Among its declared objectives are: "Verify and define the composition of botanicals"; "discover means of enhancing and accelerating the healing process beyond the effects provided by conventional medicine"; and "determine the disorders and states of wellness for which selected manipulative and body-based practices may offer meaningful benefits and specify the optimal circumstances under which the chosen manipulative and body-based practices are performed." The results of these avenues of research are as of 2007 yet to be seen.

In the following chapter, two authors debate whether NC-CAM strategic plans are providing valid and worthwhile research data. The NCCAM's former director, Stephen Straus, and his deputy director, Margaret Chesney, contend that the center is providing a vital service by helping consumers make more informed decisions about alternative medicine. Physician and critic Kimball Atwood IV, however, believes the tepid results of the first five-year plan illustrate that the NCCAM is a waste of taxpayers' money. Whether the views of Atwood and other critics like him will ultimately succeed in abolishing the institution is unknown as of 2007, but these viewpoints along with the others in this chapter reveal the controversy surrounding government involvement in the regulation and research of alternative medicine.

| "We must acknowledge that herbal supplements are drugs and should be regulated as such."

The FDA Should Tightly Regulate Herbal Supplements

Joe Dobrin

In the following viewpoint, Joe Dobrin argues that the U.S. Food and Drug Administration (FDA) should impose strict regulations upon herbal supplements. Because some of these supplements have proven dangerous, Dobrin maintains that the FDA needs to ensure the public of the purity and safety of all herbal products. In order to do this, Dobrin states, the FDA must have the enforcement powers to regulate herbal supplements in the same manner that it regulates other drugs.

As you read, consider the following questions:

1. As Dobrin relates, what have been the dangerous properties of yohimbine and androstenedione?
2. What does Dobrin claim are the two reasons that regulatory enforcement of supplements is currently ineffectual?

Joe Dobrin, "A Call to Pharms: The Need for Tighter FDA Regulation of the Neutraceutical Industry," *Mount Sinai Journal of Medicine*, vol. 73, no. 2, March 2006, pp. 565–66. Copyright © 2006 Mount Sinai Journal of Medicine. This material is used by permission of John Wiley & Sons, Inc.

3. What "loophole" in the FDA regulatory guidelines does Dobrin say supplement makers exploit in marketing their products?

Beverly Hames sought a natural remedy for her persistent backaches. She visited an acupuncturist, who gave her a list of Chinese herbal preparations, some of which contained aristolochic acid. Two years later her kidneys began to fail. She ultimately received a kidney transplant and must now take anti-rejection medication for the rest of her life. Only later did she learn that the sale of aristolochic acid has been banned in several European countries due to its carcinogenic properties and its association with kidney failure. The Food and Drug Administration (FDA) issued a consumer warning in 2001, but the product remains on the market in the U.S.

Unfortunately, Ms. Hames' experience, cited in the May 2004 edition of *Consumer Reports*, is not unique. Many people take herbal supplements (also known as "neutraceuticals") under the mistaken impression that they are safer than regulated pharmaceuticals because herbal remedies are "natural" and don't contain "chemicals." The herbal supplement industry exploits this ignorance by implying that substances derived from plants are safer than chemicals synthesized in a lab. In fact, however, the active ingredients in herbal supplements are chemicals.

Dangerous Substances

Although most herbal supplements are benign, some of these chemicals induce dangerous reactions in the human body. Aristolochic acid is far from the only chemical in herbal supplements currently on the market that has been associated with serious morbidity. The sexual stimulant yohimbine has been associated with heart and lung disease. The muscle-enhancing steroid androstenedione (andro), made famous by the baseball slugger Mark McGwire, increases cancer risk and decreases HDL (good) cholesterol. And kava, commonly found

The Powerful Supplement Industry

So-called "dietary supplements," such as DHEA, saw palmetto and chondroitin, present the biggest problem [with
the complementary and alternative medicine industry].

Marketers often sell them under the guise of a mom-
and-pop alternative to big pharma. Yet the $29 billion-a-
year dietary supplement industry wields such power that it
got Congress to pass a law in 1994 that basically frees it to
peddle almost anything that doesn't kill people with claims
of medical benefit that need not be proven.

Robert Bazell, "Ignoring the Failures of Alternative Medicine,"
MSNBC.com, *October 25, 2006. www.msnbc.msn.com.*

in energy drinks, is associated with liver damage. Although the
FDA has recently issued warnings about the use of all of these
chemicals, none has been banned from the market.

A Lack of Effective Regulation

Unlike prescription drugs regulated by the FDA, there are no
standards of quality or purity for neutraceuticals. This is because they are considered food additives, and as such, they are
not subject to the much stricter drug regulatory authority of
the FDA. There have been periodic calls for reform from medical and consumer protection groups. Unfortunately, these actions have achieved only a modicum of legislative success.

The central piece of legislation regulating herbal supplement neutraceuticals is the 1994 Dietary Supplement Health
and Education Act (DSHEA). Although this law aimed to reduce the number of unsafe herbal supplements on the market,
in practice it has had very little effect. Standing the drug regulation paradigm on its head, this act requires the FDA to
demonstrate that a supplement is *unsafe* before it can ban it
from the market, rather than placing the burden of establish-

ing safety and efficacy on the supplement makers. As a result, the FDA takes on only the most demonstrably dangerous products, and even then the process often takes years.

Poor Enforcement

Inadequate regulatory authority is not the only problem. Enforcement is hamstrung for two major reasons. First, authority is split between the FDA, which is charged with maintaining the safety of neutraceuticals, and the Federal Trade Commission (FTC), which ostensibly prohibits manufacturers from making unsupported claims of efficacy when advertising their products. In practice, lack of communication between these agencies has allowed many manufacturers to imply their products are effective without rigorous scientific testing to back up their claims. Second, neither of these agencies is adequately staffed or funded to achieve its mission. For example, the FDA's supplement division has a budget of $10 million and employs 60 people to regulate a $20 billion-a-year industry. By contrast, Congress recently appropriated $515 million to fund nearly 3,000 employees of the FDA's Center for Drug Evaluation and Research to regulate the pharmaceutical industry, whose annual sales are only 12 times the amount of supplement sales. It is little wonder that only a few dozen actions have been brought against supplement makers over the last decade.

Making Largely Unsupported Claims

The FDA's 2005 *Dietary Supplement Labeling Guide*, promulgated in April of 2005, has largely been a disappointment to reformers. The *Guide* intends that health claims made by herbal manufacturers be subject to much stricter standards. In theory, a neutraceutical manufacturer that wants to claim its product cures cancer must get prior approval from the FDA, and the claim must be supported by a consensus of the scientific literature. However, there is a large loophole. The FDA allows manufacturers to make "qualified claims" that require neither FDA approval nor a scientific consensus. They must merely cite *any* scientific study that supports their claim, and add a disclaimer (perhaps in fine print) that there is no scientific consensus about this finding. It is not difficult to imagine manufacturers citing obscure studies, potentially even from industry-funded labs, to meet this requirement.

Lest the industry miss the message that nothing has changed, the new guidelines are voluntary. As the guide says, "This guidance represents the Food and Drug Administration's (FDA's) current thinking on the topic. It does not create or confer any rights for or on any person and does not operate to bind [the] FDA or the public. You can use an alternative approach if the approach satisfies the requirements of the applicable statutes and regulations."

Time for Reform

It is time to change the way the FDA regulates herbal supplements. We must acknowledge that herbal supplements are drugs and should be regulated as such. The risks of not doing so will only increase.

Regulatory reform would place the onus on neutraceutical manufacturers to establish the safety and efficacy of their products. Only after subjecting these products to rigorous clinical trials to substantiate their claims should these products be allowed on the market, and then only with clear labeling of appropriate dosing and contraindications. To maximize compliance, enforcement should be centralized in only one agency—the drug regulatory division of the FDA, with significantly higher staffing and funding levels than the supplements division. By placing regulatory authority under the aegis of a division with teeth, the prognosis for future Beverly Hameses should be much brighter.

| "It is a larger understanding of the proper use of herbs that should shape our public policy about dietary supplements."

Tighter Regulation of Herbal Supplements May Overshadow Their Appropriate Use

James S. Gordon

In the following viewpoint, James S. Gordon uses the Food and Drug Administration's (FDA) decision to ban the herbal supplement ephedra as an example of a policy decision with problematic consequences. Although Gordon agrees that the supplement—as improperly prescribed—warranted FDA restriction, he maintains that it is the misuse and misunderstanding of herbal supplements that gives these valuable medicines a bad reputation in the medical field. Gordon does not believe more regulation of herbs is needed; rather he asserts that using the regulatory tools already in place coupled with an open mind toward the proper use of herbal supplements will prove that natural medicines are an asset to the healing profession. Gordon is a professor

*at Georgetown University Medical School in Washington, D.C.,
and a former chair of the White House Commission on Complementary and Alternative Medicine Policy.*

As you read, consider the following questions:

1. According to Gordon, what ailments has ephedra been
   used to counteract in traditional practices?
2. In Gordon's estimatation, what percentage of Americans
   may be using herbal supplements and other alternative
   approaches?
3. What did Gordon and the Commission on Complementary and Alternative Medicine Policy suggest the FDA do
   to better implement the full powers at its discretion?

The Food and Drug Administration (FDA) has recently issued a ban on the dietary supplement ephedra because it
poses "an unreasonable risk for the public health." The ban,
which was front-page news when it was first announced, is
sensible and necessary. The action may, however, obscure
some of the larger issues related to the public's use of dietary
supplements and frustrate rather than further their more intelligent integration into healthcare.

The ban is necessary because ephedra, used as an aid to
weight loss and energy enhancement, has been implicated in
the cardiac deaths of scores, perhaps hundreds, of mostly
young Americans, and in the "adverse events"—strokes, heart
attacks, fainting, anxiety—of many more. It is necessary because the companies that have profited hugely from manufacturing these supplements have long ignored or rationalized
these dreadful consequences.

The Politics of Banning Ephedra

Proponents of strict regulation, including many editorialists,
regard ephedra as Exhibit A, the most obviously damaging of
what they expect to be a succession of dangerous dietary

The 10 Most Common Herbal Medicines

- Gingko biloba

- St. John's Wort

- Echinacea

- Ginseng

- Garlic

- Saw Palmetto

- Kava-kava

- Valerian

- Milk Thistle

- Feverfew

Brent A. Bauer,
"Herbal Medicine: The Good, the Bad, and the Ugly,"
SoCRA Source, August 2003, pp. 27–30.

supplements that will need to be outlawed. Scrap the Dietary Supplement and Health Education Act of 1994 (DSHEA), they demand, so the public will no longer have easy access to these products. Many manufacturers and health food store owners consider ephedra's case to be exceptional: The herb is the dangerous pariah whose obvious misconduct is a stark contrast to the good behavior of other natural substances.

The truth, however, is far more complex, as is a more intelligent and comprehensive approach to the use of herbs and other dietary supplements.

Ephedra (known in China as *ma huang*) has been used therapeutically for thousands of years. The first written account of its properties appeared in *The Divine Husbandman's*

Materia Medica some 2,000 years ago. Both ancient Chinese practitioners and modern Western scientists have observed its efficacy in treating asthma, in raising abnormally low blood pressure, promoting diuresis (the loss of excess fluid) and producing sweating in people with viral illnesses.

When used by traditional herbalists, ephedra's dosage is carefully calibrated to the individual patient and his or her needs. Almost always, it is used in combination with other herbs, which enhance therapeutic effects and balance potential side effects. It is most definitely not used for weight loss or performance enhancement. In fact, the elevated metabolism, fast heart rate, and hyperalert state that are regarded as benefits by those who sell and use ephedra for weight loss, are considered by experienced herbalists to be signs of toxic and potentially dangerous overdosing.

How to Address the Problem

The reasons why ephedra is now being banned have nothing to do with its real therapeutic value and its appropriate use. This last point is extremely important. It is the deliberate misunderstanding of the traditional use of herbs and the irresponsible exploitation for economic gain which have compelled the FDA to act. And it is a larger understanding of the proper use of herbs that should shape our public policy about dietary supplements.

In using herbs and other traditional approaches, such as meditation, guided imagery, dietary therapies, and acupuncture, Americans in large numbers (perhaps 40% of the population) are manifesting their desire to take a more active role in their own care: to use approaches which are freer of side effects than drugs; and, especially in the case of herbs and other natural therapies, to participate in healing systems that reassert our connection with nature and value her bounty.

Banning ephedra does not ensure either greater public responsibility or more thoughtful professional and public use of herbal supplements. This requires a broader approach, which was addressed in detail by the White House Commission on Complementary and Alternative Medicine Policy, which I chaired, in a March 2002 Final Report.

Using the Regulatory Tools Already Available

The Commission specifically pointed out that the FDA was not yet using the full powers given to it by the DSHEA, including its ability to order the withdrawal of demonstrably dangerous substances. This the FDA has finally done with ephedra products. We also recommended important next steps: more effective reporting of adverse events by supplement companies to the FDA and better communication of these events by the FDA to all manufacturers and to the public: hiring by the FDA of experts in both traditional herbalism and research methods; and significantly greater monitoring of potentially fraudulent claims for supplements by the Federal Trade Commission.

There is a need, we said, for authoritative and unbiased information about these products to be available to all Americans in an easily accessible, comprehensible form, so that everyone can make informed, as well as free, choices about natural products. We suggested this could be one of the functions of a Coordinating Office on Integrative Medicine at the level of the Secretary of Health and Human Services. We also urged full disclosure, at the point of sale, in the form, for example, of package inserts (modeled on those that accompany prescription drugs) of what is known scientifically about the benefits, potential interactions and possible dangers of all products that are sold. None of this has been done.

More broadly, the White House Commission recommended that all health professionals be educated in the traditional systems of healing their patients are looking to—in their philosophy, as well as the scientific evidence for their practices—so they can knowledgeably counsel patients on the appropriate use, and warn them against the abuse, of natural products.

The terrible mistakes we as a society have made with ephedra will, I hope, become deeply instructive. We need to implement the laws we already have on the books, including DSHEA; to encourage—in our policies and our practices—thoughtful therapeutic use of herbs and other supplements, as well as to protect the public against dangerous exploitation, so we can all reap the benefits that nature offers us.

> "The NCCAM [National Center for Complementary and Alternative Medicine] was created by a few advocates who believed in implausible or disproved health claims. . . ."

The National Center for Complementary and Alternative Medicine Promotes Pseudoscience

Kimball C. Atwood IV

In the following viewpoint, Dr. Kimball C. Atwood IV argues that the National Center for Complementary and Alternative Medicine is an unnecessary part of the National Institutes of Health. Atwood states that the organization promotes unproven medical treatments, wasting research funds and possibly exploiting patients who submit to these unscientific practices. Atwood claims the existence of the center is perpetuated not through need of its research but because of the lobbying efforts of alternative medicine practitioners who seek legitimacy for their faulty therapies. Dr. Atwood is an anesthesiologist at the Newton-

Wellesley Hospital in Newton, Massachusetts. He is also an assistant clinical professor at the Tufts University School of Medicine and a contributing editor of the Scientific Review of Alternative Medicine.

As you read, consider the following questions:

1. What is the practice of Therapeutic Touch, as Atwood defines it?

2. In Atwood's view, why are alternative medicine clinical trials unethical?

3. Who is Ralph Moss, and why is Atwood skeptical of his credentials?

The National Center for Complementary and Alternative Medicine (NCCAM) was established in 1998, seven years after the creation of its predecessor, the Office of Alternative Medicine (OAM). The OAM had been formed not because of any medical or scientific need, but because Iowa senator Tom Harkin and former Iowa representative Berkeley Bedell believed in implausible health claims as a result of their own experiences. Bedell thought that "Naessens Serum" had cured his prostate cancer and that cow colostrum had cured his Lyme disease. He recommended "alternative medicine" to his friend Harkin, who subsequently came to believe that bee pollen had cured his hay fever.

Political wrangling, but little science, marked the history of the organization throughout the 1990s. Although the OAM was officially a part of the National Institutes of Health (NIH), it was managed more by "Harkinites" than by scientists. *Science* magazine recounted a 1993 congressional hearing held by Harkin, with Bedell as a witness:

NIH, Bedell said, should hire staffers to locate anyone who claims to have a successful therapy, search the files, and "just simply find out whether what he claims is correct."

[Subsequent to the hearing] Bedell brushed aside questions about how his field studies could be designed to avoid bias. This is a technical detail, Bedell said, and "I'm not a scientist." But he insisted at the hearing—and still insists—that field studies can be done quickly and easily, without fancy statistics or double-blinded controls.

The creation of the NCCAM as an "NIH Center" in 1998, followed by the appointment of Stephen Straus as its director in 1999, marked a noticeable change. Straus is the first director of the OAM/NCCAM to have legitimate qualifications as a biomedical scientist. He promised [in a 1999 press release] "to explore CAM [complementary and alternative medicine] healing practices in the context of rigorous science, to educate and train CAM researchers and to disseminate authoritative information about CAM to the public". Three years later he felt confident enough to tell *The Scientist*, regarding scientific opinions of the NCCAM, "I think there's very little skepticism left".

[However] in spite of Dr. Straus's convictions, the NCCAM continues to be committed more to pseudoscience and CAM advocacy than to rigorous science. . . .

Suspect Research

The NCCAM funds several "research centers," among which is Bastyr University. Another is the Center for Frontier Medicine in Biofield Science. "Biofield," according to an OAM publication, is defined as "'a massless field' that: (a) is not necessarily electromagnetic, (b) surrounds and permeates living bodies, (c) affects the body, and (d) possibly is related to qi [a spiritual energy, as defined in traditional Chinese philosophy]." According to the NCCAM Web site, "This Center facilitates and integrates research on the effects of low energy fields. The research is focused on developing standardized bioassays (cellular biology) and psychophysiological and biophysical markers of biofield effects, and on the application of the markers developed to measure outcomes in the recovery of surgical patients."

The center's principal investigator is psychologist Gary Schwartz, a colleague of alternative medicine guru Andrew Weil at the University of Arizona. Schwartz has published a book [titled *The Afterlife Experiments*] in which he claims to have shown scientifically that "consciousness continues after death" and that mediums, including [television spiritualist] John Edward, can communicate with the dead. A [2003 *Skeptical Inquirer*] critique of Schwartz's methods found them to be flawed in the most elementary of ways, such that no competent scientist could take his conclusions seriously.

Another NCCAM-sponsored research center will study "the effect of Therapeutic Touch on bone metabolism and on fibroblast biology, . . . on bone metabolism in postmenopausal women with wrist fractures and . . . the effect of healing touch on immune function in advanced cervical cancer" ([according to the] NCCAM Web site). Therapeutic Touch consists of the waving of hands several inches from a patient. Its putative basis is a manipulable "human energy field" that can be detected by practitioners but not by any scientific instrument. In experiments, however, Therapeutic Touch practitioners have failed to detect the "energy field" when denied visual cues.

Much of the rest of the research agenda of the NCCAM, such as "cranial osteopathy" for otitis media [an inflammation of the inner ear], "in Vitro Investigation of Distant Qi Gong," "Gonzalez Therapy" for cancer of the pancreas (coffee enemas, pancreatic enzymes, hundreds of daily dietary supplement pills, and hair analyses), magnets for various purposes, acupuncture for diarrhea in HIV patients, and oral shark cartilage for cancer, is either so implausible as to not warrant spending public monies or has already been disproved in other settings. Some trials appear to employ more than one method in the same study group, ensuring that even if an effect exists there will be no way to tell what caused it.

A few of the trials and research centers seem, on their face, to be legitimate. Examples of these are the Glucosamine/

Congress Should Stop Funding Alternative Medicine

Special commercial interests and irrational, wishful thinking created NCCAM. NCCAM is the only entity in the NIH [National Institutes of Health] devoted to an ideological approach to health. To correct the situation, Congress must consider at least interrupting funding of NCCAM while results of work in progress mature. NCCAM could be dissolved, its functions returned to other NIH centers, with no loss of knowledge, and an economic gain. Funds could be invested into studies of how such misadventures into "alternative" medicine can be avoided, and on studying the warping of human perceptions and beliefs that led to the present situation. More public money for investigating methods with negligible promise is foolish economics and even more, is unwise public policy.

Wallace Sampson, "The Alternative Universe,"
Tech Central Station, December 9, 2002.
http://geomag.gfdi.fsu.edu/tss-copa/nccam_critique.html.

Chondroitin Arthritis Intervention Trial and the NCCAM's own Division of Intramural Research.

Several grants go to medical schools for the purpose of establishing "integrative medicine" centers, which begs the question of why this should be done in the absence of evidence that "integrative medicine" works. . . .

Ethical Concerns of Human Trials

Clinical trials of CAM methods pose particular ethical problems. Drawing from the primary ethics literature of the past fifty years, Ezekiel Emanuel and colleagues have proposed seven universal criteria for determining if a human study is ethical: value, scientific validity, fair subject selection, favorable risk-benefit ratio, independent review by unaffiliated individuals, informed consent, and respect for enrolled subjects. All criteria must be met in order to make such research ethical.

Highly implausible or impossible methods, such as homeopathy, craniosacral therapy, "psychic (distant) healing," Therapeutic Touch, EDTA chelation for atherosclerosis, the chiropractic "subluxation theory" and many other CAM claims are what Emanuel and colleagues refer to as "trifling hypotheses." Human studies of such methods are, a priori, unethical, quite apart from any political impetus to conduct them. This is both because of the exploitation of subjects for questions that lack "scientific or clinical value" and because such research is a waste of resources: "Comparing relative value is integral to determinations of funding priorities when allocating limited funds among alternative research proposals" [Emanuel and colleagues state in a 2000 *Journal of the American Medical Association* article]. In particular, one might add, if those funds are public. Thus the current federal allocation of $110 million per year for the NCCAM might be weighed against the $5 million per year allocated for research on spinal muscular atrophy, a devastating childhood disease that some scientists believe would be on the verge of a therapeutic breakthrough but for want of adequate funding.

These ethical arguments are not refuted by the contention that a significant fraction of the population may wish such studies to be done, or even by the argument that demonstrating such methods ineffective will benefit society. These are the usual arguments favoring the existence of the NCCAM and CAM research programs in academic medicine, and are often made even by skeptics. . . .

Biased Oversight Councils

There are two councils charged with advising the director of the NCCAM on matters related to research funding and clinical trials: the National Advisory Council for Complementary and Alternative Medicine (NACCAM) and the Cancer Advisory Panel for Complementary and Alternative Medicine (CAPCAM). It might be expected that the membership of these councils reflects the Center's professed commitment to the rigorous, skeptical inquiry of "complementary and alternative" methods. The director, however, has no formal role in selecting the council members. The members of the NACCAM are appointed by the Secretary for Health and Human Services, with these stipulations: "Of the eighteen appointed members, twelve shall be selected from among the leading representatives . . . of the health and scientific disciplines in the area of complementary and alternative medicine. Nine of the twelve shall include practitioners licensed in one or more of the major systems with which the Center is involved" (NCCAM Charter 2000). The members of the CAPCAM are appointed by the director of the NIH, but with the requirement that "of the fifteen members, eleven shall be nonfederal," including the Chair, and "nonfederal members will be selected based on their knowledge and expertise in the fields of complementary and alternative therapeutic cancer treatments" (CAPCAM Charter 2002).

Thus it can be predicted that the councils will be biased, prima facie, in favor of the very methods that the Center is charged to submit to skeptical scrutiny. An examination of the rosters of the two councils supports this prediction. Among the NACCAM members [since 2000] were [Leanna] Standish and two other naturopaths. In 2000 one of them, Anna MacIntosh, recommended "Gerson Therapy" for cancer and multiple sclerosis. This is a regimen of "detoxification" with coffee enemas and a diet including huge quantities of juices made from fruits, vegetables, and raw calf's liver. The National Cancer Institute had evaluated Gerson's claims in 1947 and again in 1959, and found them to be baseless.

The third naturopath on the NACCAM is Konrad Kail, who explains "patient-centered care" this way: "If I see a patient who has pain in his arms because his neck is out of alignment, I explain to them that we can do spinal adjustments, acupuncture, homeopathy, or we can do all three. Then I wait for their [sic] choice" [*Naturopathic Medicine*, 1997].

Another recent member of the NACCAM is Marilyn J. Schlitz, reported by skeptic Dr. Tim Gorski [in a 2001 response to a statement by U.S. Representative Dan Burton] to be "an astral voyager 'remote viewer' who was praised by Russell Targ for having 'achieved the greatest statistical significance of any remote-viewing experiment so far conducted' in exploring tourist sites in Rome from her home in Detroit, Michigan". . . .

On the CAPCAM still sits Ralph Moss, one of the original "Harkinites." His *Cancer Chronicles* newsletter has suggested that homeopathy and other implausible treatments can cure cancer. He has also accused the Mayo Clinic of being "fraudulent" [in a 1993 edition of his newsletter] because of its study that demonstrated the ineffectiveness of laetrile [an almond extract that some claim fights cancer]. This exposes the fallacy of the social usefulness of studies that disprove sectarian methods. . . .

An Unneeded, Unhelpful Organization

Straus has written that the NCCAM "was created to foster and build a research enterprise that subjects complementary and alternative medicine to open-minded, hypothesis-driven investigation". That is inaccurate. The NCCAM was created by a few advocates who believed in implausible or disproved health claims, including laetrile, and who felt that the scientific "establishment" was unfairly suppressing them. As such, the Center's role has been more one of advocacy than of science. Calls for its abolition have been reasoned and comprehensive.

After more than ten years and $200 million, OAM/ NCCAM-sponsored research has not demonstrated efficacy for any CAM method, nor has the Center informed the public that any method is useless. It continues to fund and promote pseudoscience. It continues to be influenced by powerful ideologues.

The problem with so-called Complementary and Alternative Medicine, in a nutshell, is that it is an assortment of implausible, dishonest, expensive, and sometimes dangerous claims that are exuberantly promoted to a scientifically naïve public. The NCCAM, so far, has not been part of the solution.

> *"The public is using [complementary and alternative medicines] without proof of efficacy or safety, which is the very reason that NCCAM-funded research is so important."*

The National Center for Complementary and Alternative Medicine Promotes Valuable Research

Stephen E. Straus and Margaret A. Chesney

The National Center for Complementary and Alternative Medicine (NCCAM) is a valuable research institution, argue Stephen E. Straus and Margaret A. Chesney in the following viewpoint. According to the authors, the NCCAM has worked with mainstream medicine authorities to analyze the effects of alternative medicines and to ensure that these medicines are safe for consumers. The organization establishes rigorous safeguards to test complementary and alternative medicines (CAM) and is as eager as CAM's critics to discard those treatments that have no health benefit or are harmful. Stephen E. Straus was the director of the NCCAM from 1999 (following NCCAM's inception in

Stephen E. Straus and Margaret A. Chesney, "Enhanced: In Defense of NCCAM," *Science*, vol. 313, no. 5785, July 21, 2006, pp. 303–304. Copyright 2006 by AAAS. Reproduced by permission.

1998) until his resignation in 2007. Margaret A. Chesney is NCCAM's first deputy director and leads the Division of Extramural Research and Training.

As you read, consider the following questions:

1. Why did Congress found NCCAM, according to Straus and Chesney?

2. As the authors state, why does the Food and Drug Administration not regulate dietary supplements as stringently as dietary drugs?

3. What do the authors cite as some of the beneficial research the NCCAM has produced since its inception?

The National Center for Complementary and Alternative Medicine (NCCAM) is one of the 27 institutes and centers that constitute the National Institutes of Health (NIH). Its mission is to investigate complementary and alternative medicine (CAM) in the context of rigorous science, to train CAM researchers, and to disseminate authoritative information to the public and professional communities. From its beginning, NCCAM has encountered controversy and strong sentiments for and against the scientific study of CAM. . . . Some criticisms have been valid and have led to more stringent policies on product quality and safety, for example. Others are misinformed. Our goal is to bring fact and clarity to this discussion, just as we seek to bring science to the assessment of CAM.

History of Establishing NCCAM

The U.S. Congress established NCCAM in 1998 to bring scientific rigor to studies of CAM by the same legislative process used to establish other NIH institutes and centers. This is a challenging mandate, one that required establishing a new CAM research enterprise that met the high standards of biomedical research for which NIH is known. NCCAM has outlined its approach to studying CAM in its 5-year strategic plans, the most recent of which was published in 2005. These plans were developed with balanced debate and advice from a wide range of individuals representing the scientific community, conventional and CAM practitioners, and the public.

The criticism that only a handful of individuals have shaped the NCCAM agenda is not accurate. In creating our second strategic plan, NCCAM embarked on a year-long process of agenda-setting dialog. The center held a think tank of leading scholars, including three current and past NIH institute directors; convened stakeholder forums on the East and West coasts; assembled a strategic planning workshop with more than 80 individuals from mainstream medicine and CAM communities; and sought input from over 1500 individuals and professional organizations. We specifically included distinguished conventional scientists (without experience in CAM) to lend their expertise to discussions of CAM-related research challenges.

NCCAM Advisory Council and Peer Review

As with other institutes at NIH, the composition of the NCCAM Advisory Council was specified in congressional language. The council includes individuals with conventional scientific and medical training, such as M.D.'s and Ph.D.'s, and others with CAM expertise, as well as representatives from the lay public. NCCAM's Advisory Council has scientists with exemplary records of accomplishment in a variety of disciplines. This balanced composition reflects NIH's interdisciplinary approach to today's complex scientific questions. The 17 current council members have published 414 peer-reviewed articles and received 35 NIH grants in the period from 2001 to 2006 (23 of which were awarded by other NIH institutes).

NCCAM's peer-review process is the same as other NIH institutes, i.e., content experts review applications in their area of expertise. Cardiologists review applications on ischemic

Important Events in NCCAM History

October 1991—The U.S. Congress passes legislation (P.L. 102–170) that provides $2 million in funding for fiscal year 1992 to establish the Office of Alternative Medicine (OAM), an office within the National Institutes of Health (NIH) to investigate and evaluate promising unconventional medical practices.

September 1993—The first OAM research project grants are funded through the National Center for Research Resources.

December 1993—The Alternative Medicine Program Advisory Council is established.

October 1998—NCCAM is established by Congress under the Omnibus Appropriations Act of 1999 (P.L. 105–277). This bill amends Title IV of the Public Health Service Act and elevates the status of the OAM to an NIH Center.

May 1999—NCCAM independently awards its first research project grant.

August 1999—The National Advisory Council on Complementary and Alternative Medicine (NACCAM) is chartered.

October 1999—Stephen E. Straus, M.D., is appointed the first Director of NCCAM.

February 2001—NCCAM and the National Library of Medicine launch *CAM on PubMed*, a comprehensive Internet source of research-based information on Complementary and Alternative Medicine (CAM).

April 2002—Results of NCCAM's first clinical trial, of St. John's wort for major depression, are released.

May 2004—NCCAM and the National Center for Health Statistics (NCHS) of the Centers for Disease Control and Prevention (CDC) announce the release of the largest, most comprehensive, and most reliable survey findings to date on Americans' use of CAM.

January 2005—NCCAM publishes the strategic plan, *Expanding Horizons of Health Care: Strategic Plan 2005–2009*, following a year-long process of input from the public, staff, and groups of outside experts.

U.S. Department of Health and Human Services,
"National Center for Complementary and Alternative Medicine,"
National Institutes of Health,, *June 21, 2007.*
www.nih.gov/about/almanac/organization/NCCAM.htm.

heart disease, and pharmacologists, including pharmacognosists, review applications on botanical products. NCCAM's
investigator-initiated R01 grant applications are reviewed by
study sections convened by the NIH Center for Scientific Review; thus, they compete on an even playing field with all
other applications to NIH. All members of NIH peer-review
panels and advisory councils, including those at NCCAM, adhere to NIH policies concerning conflict of interest. The NC-
CAM Advisory Council acts as a second level of review.

Product Quality and Patient Safety

One of the most challenging issues in studying CAM has been
the quality of dietary supplement products available for research and the variability of quality and content of products
in the marketplace. Unlike pharmaceutical firms, dietary
supplement manufacturers do not have to establish efficacy
before marketing their products to the public. The Food and
Drug Administration (FDA) regulates dietary supplements as
foods, not drugs. Therefore, FDA does not analyze the content
of dietary supplements. Moreover, U.S. law does not define
the term "standardized." Thus, product quality and consistency can vary. This is a challenge for both researchers and the
public.

NCCAM has developed a multifaceted strategy to ensure
the quality of biologically active agents used in NCCAM-
supported research. Now, before NCCAM funds a project, a
Product Quality Working Group, composed of pharmacologists, pharmacognosists, and other scientists, reviews information to determine whether the product is of the quality required to replicate research findings. Information is collected
on more than 20 factors, including product characterization,
standardization, contamination, consistency, and stability, that
could affect the quality of research data. NCCAM also carries
out quality-control assessments of random samples of biologi-

cally active products that are being used in the studies it funds. The selected samples are sent to independent laboratories for analysis, thus providing information on stability, quality, and characterization.

In addition to these product-quality measures, NCCAM has also established an independent phase I resource center to conduct preclinical pharmacology research on dietary supplements. In selecting candidate supplements for study, NCCAM places a priority on products that are widely used by the public, yet have insufficient data on factors such as dose range, bioequivalence, pharmacokinetics, bioavailability, and botanical-drug interaction—information that is currently lacking for many botanical products.

The safety of individuals participating in NCCAM-supported clinical studies is of paramount importance to the center. In addition to NIH-required safeguards for human subject protection, NCCAM has an Office of Clinical and Regulatory Affairs to provide oversight of NCCAM studies involving human subjects. This office oversees the Data and Safety Monitoring Boards for NCCAM's clinical trials and ensures compliance with Institutional Review Boards' guidance and FDA regulations. Other NIH institutes have similar offices. This research infrastructure has been created to ensure that the research that NCCAM funds will be reproducible and meet the rigorous standards expected by NIH-funded research.

NCCAM Research

In the early years of NCCAM, there was a sense of urgency to scientifically assess a range of CAM therapies that had been in long use by the public in the absence of proof of safety or efficacy. Thus, NCCAM undertook a number of clinical trials in its first years, many with support from other NIH institutes. In doing so, we have gained valuable experience that has informed our thinking about challenging issues in CAM research such as dosing, methodology, and other experimental factors.

When early trials of botanical products, such as saw palmetto, did not show efficacy, NCCAM focused attention on the doses used in these studies, which were based on those widely used by the public. NCCAM now has a policy of requiring dose-range studies and other preclinical research before conducting clinical trials. The NCCAM research portfolio now includes more basic research focused on mechanisms of action, pharmacokinetics of herbal products, drug-herb interactions, and dose optimization, as well as clinical effects. This shift is reflected in the decline of the NCCAM clinical research portfolio from 80% in 2000 to 68% in 2005. The balance of basic and clinical research continues to serve the specific public health issues that NCCAM was created to address.

Contrary to the criticism that NCCAM prescribes areas of study to investigators, the center, like other NIH institutes, accepts unsolicited, investigator-initiated applications that are based on ideas formulated by the applicant, not NCCAM. The percentage of solicited grants funded by year varies, but in the last three fiscal years [2003–2005], about 87% of NCCAM-funded grants were unsolicited. NCCAM welcomes well-designed research applications on a wide range of CAM therapies.

Research Findings

In 2002, the National Health Interview Survey of more than 31,000 people found that 62% of Americans use some form of CAM. The public is using CAM without proof of efficacy or safety, which is the very reason that NCCAM-funded research is so important.

NCCAM's research has provided valuable information on the physiologic pathway of the placebo effect using state-of-the-art brain imaging technologies, the efficacy of acupuncture to relieve pain associated with osteoarthritis of the knee, and a potential role for glucosamine-chondroitin for patients with moderate-to-severe osteoarthritis pain. NCCAM's research is in the forefront of understanding the interactions of prescription drugs and dietary supplements. NCCAM's scrutiny of product safety informed the FDA's decision to withdraw ephedra from the marketplace.

These are a few examples of the more than 1,000 peer-reviewed publications that have resulted from the first 7 years of basic and clinical research supported by NCCAM. NCCAM's research results will help build a fuller understanding of what CAM can offer. We not only expand our knowledge about the tested therapy but also learn more about the condition it is meant to treat. Overall, we should regard each study's results in the same way—as yet another crucial piece of the research puzzle.

Working with the Medical Community

After only 7 years, NCCAM has made important contributions in a field that is fraught with controversy and challenges. NCCAM is applying the same scientific standards to the conduct of research and its review as used by other NIH institutes. We have raised the bar on the study design and methods used in CAM research, including the quality of products under investigation. Our portfolio of basic research will inform subsequent clinical studies to ensure that we are testing a high-quality product, at the optimal dose, and in the appropriate population.

Before the establishment of NCCAM, there was no central source of CAM information. NCCAM brings evidence-based information on CAM to the public, practitioners, and researchers. NCCAM disseminates research findings and provides reliable information about commonly used CAM practices through numerous channels, including its information clearinghouse and its award-winning Web site. NCCAM's communications program deals with a field that is controversial, that has many critics, and that reaches a public that wants reliable information.

We fully support the Institute of Medicine's recommendation that the same principles and standards of evidence apply to all treatments, whether labeled as conventional medicine or CAM. We believe that we have succeeded in establishing a research enterprise that will achieve this standard. While challenges remain, we are confident that knowledge gained from NACCAM-supported studies will continue to inform the public, health-care providers, and policy-makers about how and when evidence-based CAM therapies should be used and effectively integrated into conventional medical care.

Periodical Bibliography

The following articles have been selected to supplement the diverse views presented in this chapter.

Mike Adams
"The Big Vitamin Scare: American Medical Association Claims Vitamins May Kill You," *NewsTarget.com*, May 28, 2007. www.newstarget.com.

Edzard Ernst
"Regulation of Complementary and Alternative Medicine," *Focus on Alternative and Complementary Therapies*, September 2003.

Ruiping Fan
"Modern Western Science as a Standard for Traditional Chinese Medicine: A Critical Appraisal," *Journal of Law, Medicine, & Ethics*, Summer 2003.

Thomas Fields-Meyer, Carol Guensburg, Susan Keating
"Should He Be Forced to Have Chemo?" *People*, August 21, 2006.

Phil B. Fontanarosa, Drummond Rennie, Catherine D. DeAngelis
"The Need for Regulation of Dietary Supplements—Lessons from Ephedra," *JAMA: Journal of the American Medical Association*, March 26, 2003.

David J. Hufford
"Evaluating Complementary and Alternative Medicine: The Limits of Science and Scientists," *Journal of Law, Medicine, & Ethics*, Summer 2003.

Marilynn Larkin
"Alternative Medicine Centre Aims for Mainstream Status," *Lancet*, August 18, 2001.

Donald M. Marcus and Arthur P. Grollman
"Review for NCCAM Is Overdue," *Science*, July 21, 2006.

Nicholas Zamiska
"Dueling Therapies: Is a Shotgun Better than a Silver Bullet?" *Wall Street Journal*, March 2, 2007.

For Further Discussion

Chapter 1

1. Dana Ullman repeatedly mentions that homeopathic therapies are prescribed based on a patient's physical and mental symptoms. Robert Todd Carroll concedes that homeopathic remedies may have some value because they have a psychological component that eases the patient's mind, which may in turn aid the body's own healing mechanisms. Although the two authors agree that homeopathic treatments have a potentially useful mental component, how do their arguments diverge to show opposing views of homeopathy's effectiveness? In drafting your answer, consider Ullman's statement, "One of the special features of homeopathy is that whenever a patient is given a homeopathic medicine that does not match his or her symptoms, nothing happens." How does Ullman see this "special feature" as a strength of homeopathy; how would Carroll likely frame this as one of homeopathy's weaknesses?

2. Although John Jackson dismisses chiropractic theories and treatments as ineffectual (even dangerous), Michael Menke tells his readers, "If you have pain that is not improving with your current self-care or treatment strategies, or you have a problem specifically related to your back, neck or spine, see if chiropractic can help." Do you agree with Menke's statement? Would you seek (or have you sought) the services of a chiropractor? Explain why or why not and be sure to refer to the arguments in the viewpoints.

3. Danny Siegenthaler argues that pharmaceutical companies are investigating the curative properties of herbs even as

they publicly dismiss the effectiveness of herbal medicines in order to maintain the sales of manufactured drugs. After reading Siegenthaler's viewpoint, do you think his assessment is accurate? Examine the reasons pharmaceutical companies might be downplaying the usefulness of herbal medicines as well as the motivation behind Siegenthaler's criticism.

Chapter 2

1. Benedict Carey and others have pointed out that people often experiment with alternative medicines because they find conventional medicine and its practitioners to be too impersonal. Do you agree that conventional health care lacks warmth and compassion? Are these essential ingredients of the healing process? How could conventional health care become more sympathetic? Be sure to be specific in your suggestions.

2. After reading the viewpoints by Carey and Goldacre, explain why you think alternative medicine is so popular today. Be sure to acknowledge which of these authors' arguments you strongly agree with and which you find less relevant. You may also propose other reasons not covered in these viewpoints.

Chapter 3

1. Timothy N. Gorski insists that medicine and religion cannot mix in conventional health care because it would be impossible for doctors to cater to every patient's religious creeds. Thus, treatments involving a religious dimension might offend some patients who either have different beliefs or hold no religious views. Barbara Anan Kogan, however, states that spirituality can be more broadly interpreted to include "an individual's sense of purpose and meaning in life beyond material values." She contends that addressing this aspect of a patient during healthcare

visits can be beneficial in healing. Do you think that discussing spirituality, as Kogan defines it, should be part of healthcare visits, or is any attempt to address the spiritual side of people apt to incur the kinds of problems Gorski mentions? Using the authors' arguments and your own, explain your thoughts on this matter.

2. After reading the viewpoints by the National Academies and E. Haavi Morreim, explain whether you think alternative medicines and treatments should be held to the same rigors and standards as conventional medicine. When giving your response, consider that, besides Morreim's arguments, some proponents of alternative medicine insist that these remedies simply do not conform to conventional ways of measurement, while others have argued that alternative medicines and treatments have been the subject of conventional tests and have successfully proven their effectiveness.

3. Philippe Szapary advocates integrating CAM into traditional medical education, while Wallace Sampson fears that if medical schools adopt CAM programs, they will legitimize the supposed effectiveness of these treatments without compelling students to critically analyze their theoretical healing value. Do you think CAM should be part of a medical education? What are the benefits or dangers of incorporating CAM more widely into the curricula?

Chapter 4

1. Joe Dobrin argues that the government should monitor herbal supplements more closely because of their potential dangers if improperly used. James S. Gordon, however, claims that, while it is necessary to ban harmful products, portraying herbal supplements as having unknown or potentially dangerous qualities in need of increased regulation will taint them in the eyes of health practitioners and

overshadow the long history of their effective use. After examining both of the authors' viewpoints, discuss whether there is a system that would satisfy both Dobrin and Gordon.

2. After reading the viewpoints by Kimball C. Atwood and Stephen E. Straus and Margaret A. Chesney, explore whether the National Center for Complementary and Alternative Medicine should exist as a government institution. If you believe the institution is legitimate, explain what value it has. If you think it needs to be abolished, explain why and address the problems that might arise in its absence. Also consider whether there is a third option that might suit the authors.

Organizations to Contact

The editors have compiled the following list of organizations concerned with the issues debated in this book. The descriptions are derived from materials provided by the organizations. All have publications or information available for interested readers. The list was compiled on the date of publication of the present volume; the information provided here may change. Be aware that many organizations take several weeks or longer to respond to inquiries, so allow as much time as possible.

Alternative Medicine Foundation
P.O. Box 60016, Potomac, MD   20859
(301) 340-1960 • fax: (301) 340-1936
Web site: www.amfoundation.org

Founded in 1998, the Alternative Medicine Foundation provides information to the public and professional spheres about complementary and alternative healthcare options and the benefits of integrative medicine. The main goals of the organization are to promote ethical integrative medicine use and ensure that indigenous therapies are not lost in the world of modern health care. The organization's Web site contains links to the information databases *HerbMed* and *TibetMed*, as well as numerous resource guides on general and specific CAM modalities.

Alternative Medicine Homepage
Charles B. Wessel, MLS, Pittsburgh, PA   15261
e-mail: cbw@pitt.edu
Web site: www.pitt.edu/~cbw/altm.html

Medical science librarian Charles B. Wessel created the Alternative Medicine Homepage at the University of Pittsburgh as a central source for alternative medicine information on the Internet. Links to databases of articles on alternative medicine, mailing lists, and government and Internet resources are all available and annotated on this site. Both pro-CAM and skeptical sites are included in the listings.

American Association for Health Freedom
4620 Lee Hwy., Suite 210, Arlington, VA   22207
(800) 230-2762 • fax: (703) 624-6380
e-mail: healthfreedom2000@yahoo.com
Web site: www.apma.net

American Association for Health Freedom (AAHF) provides advocacy on behalf of healthcare practitioners and consumers who use complementary and alternative therapies. This organization works to ensure that government regulations do not infringe on individuals' ability to choose the type of medical intervention they provide or receive. Articles on topics concerning the AAHF as well as information on current issues being pursued by the organization are available on the Web site.

American Chiropractic Association
1701 Clarendon Blvd., Arlington, VA   22209
(703) 276-8800 • fax: (703) 243-2593
e-mail: memberinfo@acatoday.org
Web site: www.amerchiro.org

The American Chiropractic Association (ACA), a professional organization for chiropractors, works to advance understanding and standards of chiropractic methods through lobbying efforts, public relations, increased research, and provision of educational materials. Publications such as *ACA News, Journal of the American Chiropractic Association (JACA) Online, Journal of Manipulative and Physiological Therapeutics (JMPT)*, and *Healthy Living Fact Sheets: Patient Education Pages* provide both professionals and patients with the opportunity to learn more about the benefits of the chiropractic modality.

American Council on Science and Health
1995 Broadway, Second Floor, New York, NY   10023-5860

(212) 362-7044 • fax: (212) 362-4919
e-mail: acsh@acsh.org
Web site: www.acsh.org

The American Council on Science and Health (ACSH) provides consumers with accurate information on health- and science-related issues. Through activities such as seminars, press conferences, and coordination with the media, ACSH is dedicated to dispensing unbiased information regarding topics such as alternative medicine, nutrition, pharmaceuticals, and tobacco. The "Facts and Fears" section of the organization's Web site provides a searchable database of articles published by the organization; additionally, the organization's other topical publications can be browsed and searched.

American Holistic Medical Association

P.O. Box 2016, Edmonds, WA   98020
(425) 967-0737 • fax: (425) 771-9588
e-mail: ahma@holisticmedicine.org
Web site: www.holisticmedicine.org

The American Holistic Medical Association (AHMA) is a professional organization of medical doctors, doctors of osteopathic medicine, and medical students who practice or are studying to practice holistic medicine. AHMA works to aid these individuals in their careers and to provide information for professionals and the public about holistic practices. Physician referrals through the organization's database as well as a guide to choosing a holistic practitioner are available on the organization's Web site.

American Medical Association

515 N. State St., Chicago, IL   60610
(800) 621-8335
Web site: www.ama-assn.org

The American Medical Association (AMA) is a professional organization of physicians that seeks to improve the health of all Americans. The organization provides policy guidelines on pertinent issues in health care and provides an opportunity for doctors to collaborate nationwide in addressing the needs of patients. Issues such as the integration of alternative medicine and the use of dietary supplements have been addressed in the pages of the AMA's publication, the *Journal of the American Medical Association (JAMA)*.

Bravewell Collaborative

1818 Oliver Ave. South, Minneapolis, MN   55405
(612) 377-8400
e-mail: donor@bravewell.org
Web site: www.bravewell.org

The Bravewell Collaborative is a philanthropic organization with the mission of increasing the use of integrative medicine in health care. With scholarship programs that encourage young medical students to enter the field of integrative medicine, public education through the production of the PBS documentary *The New Medicine*, and leadership awards, the Bravewell Collaborative has been at the forefront of promoting improved health care through the cooperation of traditional and alternative medicines. Detailed information about integrative medicine and its relationship to health care is available on the organization's Web site.

Citizens for Health

2104 Stevens Ave. South, Minneapolis, MN   55404
(612) 879-7585
e-mail: info@citizens.org
Web site: www.citizens.org

As a national consumer advocacy organization, Citizens for Health works to ensure that consumers have the opportunity and freedom to choose the type of health care they desire. Through grassroots organization and cooperation with private industry, Citizens for Health promotes the idea that government legislation should always protect the right of individuals to choose their own health services. Past issues of the newsletter, *Healthy News*, are available on the organization's Web site, as is additional information about how individuals can become involved in the Campaign for Better Health.

Committee for Skeptical Inquiry
P.O. Box 703, Amherst, NY   14226
(716) 636-1425
e-mail: info@csicop.org
Web site: www.csicop.org

The Committee for Skeptical Inquiry (CSI) is an organization dedicated to evaluating "fringe-science" claims using science-based methodology and critical inquiry. Through conferences and publications, CSI encourages skepticism about claims related to topics such as complementary and alternative medicine, as well as the paranormal, until such statements can be proven through objective study. The organization publishes the journal the *Skeptical Inquirer*, and previously published articles can be found on the CSI Web site.

Federal Trade Commission
600 Pennsylvania Ave. NW, Washington, DC   20580
(202) 326-2222
Web site: www.ftc.gov

The Federal Trade Commission (FTC) is an independent agency within the federal government that seeks to ensure that consumers in the United States receive accurate information about products and services sold to them. Projects and resources such as Operation Cure All have been commissioned by the FTC in order to increase consumer understanding and awareness on health-related claims. Articles and reports concerning complementary and alternative modalities and therapies can be found on the FTC Web site.

Food and Drug Administration
5600 Fishers Lane, Rockville, MD   20857
(888) 463-6332
Web site: www.fda.gov

The Food and Drug Administration (FDA) is the consumer protection agency of the U.S. Department of Health and Human Services that regulates the food and drug products sold to the American public. Vitamins and dietary supplements are among the products the FDA tests using science-based methods to determine their safety and efficacy. FDA ensures that labels provide information about all ingredients included in the product as well as the product's apparent risks and benefits. More detailed information about the projects of the FDA can be found on the organization's Web site.

National Center for Complementary and Alternative Medicine

9000 Rockville Pike, Bethesda, MD   20892
(888) 644-6226 • fax: (866) 464-3616
e-mail: info@nccam.nih.gov
Web site: http://nccam.nih.gov

The National Center for Complementary and Alternative Medicine (NCCAM) is the branch of the National Institute of Health (NIH) responsible for addressing issues related to complementary and alternative medicine (CAM) at the federal government level. The organization focuses on researching alternative health practices, informing professionals and the public about findings, and encouraging the integration into conventional medicine of CAM modalities that have stood up to rigorous testing and have been deemed acceptable for use. NCCAM's Web site provides access to numerous fact sheets on CAM practices, as well as video lectures and information about how to order publications.

National Council Against Health Fraud

119 Foster St., Building R, Second Floor
Peabody, MA   01960
(978) 532-9383 • fax: (978) 532-9450
e-mail: ncahf.office@verizon.net
Web site: www.ncahf.org

National Council Against Health Fraud (NCAHF) is a nonprofit consumer protection organization dedicated to providing consumers, healthcare providers, legal professionals, and legislators with accurate information on the vast variety of healthcare products and services available today. This organization works to ensure that consumers are afforded sufficient and truthful information about healthcare choices, enabling informed decision-making. NCAHF also lobbies for health-related legislation that protects consumers, and the organization publishes a free, weekly e-newsletter, *Consumer Health Digest.*

Quackwatch
P.O. Box 1747, Allentown, PA 18105
(610) 437-1795
e-mail: sbinfo@quackwatch.com
Web site: www.quackwatch.org

Quackwatch is a nonprofit corporation with the mission of exposing fraudulent practices and philosophies within the health field. Previously a member of the Consumer Federation of America, this organization strives to ensure that all claims and advertising relating to healthcare products and services are appropriately addressed and analyzed. Quackwatch is also dedicated to analyzing information dispensed on the Internet, thereby advancing the quality of information most often sought by consumers. Links to topic-specific Web sites run by the organization as well as numerous articles concerning these topics are available on the Quackwatch Web site.

The Richard and Hinda Rosenthal Center
for Complementary and Alternative Medicine
Columbia University, College of Physicians and Surgeons
New York, NY 10032
(212) 342-0101 • fax: (212) 342-0100
Web site: www.rosenthal.hs.columbia.edu

The Richard and Hinda Rosenthal Center for Complementary and Alternative Medicine is an organization within the Columbia University College of Physicians and Surgeons dedicated to applying scientific methods of testing to alternative modalities. In order to achieve the goal of a more complete integration of CAM therapies into the medical system, the center employs rigorous testing to ensure these therapies are safe and effective, educates medical professionals about the benefits of using CAM in conjunction with their practices, and provides information for medical professionals on a global scale to increase cooperation in advancing CAM practices. Information about specific CAM modalities as well as information about ongoing research can be found on the organization's Web site.

World Health Organization
Pan American Health Organization (PAHO)
Washington, DC   20037
(202) 974-3000
Web site: www.pahco.org

The World Health Organization (WHO), and its regional office, the Pan American Health Organization (PAHO), are international health organizations within the United Nations that are charged with ensuring that individuals worldwide are afforded appropriate healthcare. WHO works to achieve this goal by promulgating international health policies and programs. Because the majority of the world's populations utilize some form of alternative medicine, WHO provides information on traditional remedies and their potential health benefits. Publications such as the *WHO Global Atlas of Traditional, Complementary and Alternative Medicine* and *Legal Status of Traditional Medicine and Complementary/Alternative Medicine: A Worldwide Review* evaluate the status of traditional and CAM modalities worldwide.

Bibliography of Books

| Neil T. Anderson and Michael D. Jacobson | *The Biblical Guide to Alternative Medicine.* Ventura, CA: Regal, 2003. |

Hans Baer — *Toward an Integrative Medicine: Merging Alternative Therapies with Biomedicine.* Walnut Creek, CA: AltaMira, 2004.

Stephen Barrett and Victor Herbert — *The Vitamin Pushers: How the "Health Food" Industry Is Selling America a Bill of Goods.* Amherst, NY: Prometheus, 1994.

Stephen Barrett and William T. Jarvis, eds. — *The Health Robbers: A Close Look at Quackery in America.* Buffalo, NY: Prometheus Books, 1993.

Daniel Callahan, ed. — *The Role of Complementary and Alternative Medicine: Accommodating Pluralism.* Washington, DC: Georgetown University Press, 2002.

L. A. Chotkowski — *Chiropractic: The Greatest Hoax of the Century?* Kensington, CT: New England Books, 2002.

Michael H. Cohen — *Legal Issues in Alternative Medicine: A Guide for Clinicians, Hospitals, and Patients.* Victoria, BC, Canada: Trafford, 2003.

Committee on the Use of Complementary and Alternative Medicine by the American Public, U.S. Institute of Medicine	*Complementary and Alternative Medicine in the United States.* Washington, DC: National Academies Press, 2005.
Edzard Ernst	*Healing, Hype, or Harm? The Debate About Complementary and Alternative Medicine.* London: Hammersmith, 2007.
Daniel Eskinazi, ed.	*What Will Influence the Future of Alternative Medicine?: A World Perspective.* River Edge, NJ: World Scientific, 2001.
Bill Gray and Kenneth R. Pelletier	*Homeopathy: Science or Myth?* Berkeley, CA: North Atlantic, 2000.
Jerome Groopman	*The Anatomy of Hope: How People Prevail in the Face of Illness.* New York: Random House, 2004.
Robert D. Johnston, ed.	*The Politics of Healing: Histories of Alternative Medicine in Twentieth-Century North America.* New York: Routledge, 2004.
Harold G. Koenig, Michael E. McCullough, and David B. Larson	*Handbook of Religion and Health.* New York: Oxford University Press, 2001.

Amy L. Lansky   *Impossible Cure: The Promise of Ho-meopathy*. Portola Valley, CA: R.L. Ranch, 2003.

Christine A. Larson   *Alternative Medicine*. Westport, CT: Greenwood Press, 2006.

Michael Lenarz and Victoria St. George   *The Chiropractic Way: How Chiro-practic Care Can Stop Your Pain and Help You Regain Your Health Without Drugs or Surgery*. New York: Bantam Books, 2003.

Elizabeth R. MacKenzie and Brigit Rakel, eds.   *Complementary and Alternative Medi-cine for Older Adults: A Guide to Ho-listic Approaches to Healthy Aging*. New York: Springer, 2006.

Toby Murcott   *The Whole Story: Alternative Medicine on Trial?* New York: Macmillan, 2005.

Kenneth R. Pelletier   *The Best Alternative Medicine: What Works? What Does Not?* New York: Simon & Schuster, 2000.

James Randi   *The Faith Healers*. Buffalo, NY: Prometheus, 1987.

Alan M. Rees, ed.   *The Complementary and Alternative Medicine Information Source Book*. Westport, CT: Oryx, 2001.

Paul C. Reisser, Dale Mabe, and Robert Velarde   *Examining Alternative Medicine: An Inside Look at the Benefits and Risks*. Downers Grove, IL: InterVarsity Press, 2001.

Byron J. Richards *Fight for Your Health: Exposing the FDA's Betrayal of America.* Minneapolis, MN: Truth in Wellness, 2006.

Wallace Sampson and Lewis Vaughn, eds. *Science Meets Alternative Medicine: What the Evidence Says About Unconventional Treatments.* Amherst, NY: Prometheus, 2000.

Edward L. Schneider and Leigh Ann Hirschman *What Your Doctor Hasn't Told You and the Health-Store Clerk Doesn't Know: The Truth About Alternative Treatments and What Works.* New York: Avery, 2006.

John W. Spencer and Joseph J. Jacobs, eds. *Complementary and Alternative Medicine: An Evidence-Based Approach.* St. Louis, MO: Mosby, 2003.

Ray D. Strand with Donna K. Wallace *What Your Doctor Doesn't Know About Nutritional Medicine May Be Killing You.* Nashville, TN: Tomas Nelson, 2002.

Philip Tovey, Gary Easthope, and Jon Adams, eds. *The Mainstreaming of Complementary and Alternative Medicine: Studies in Social Context.* New York: Routledge, 2004.

Christopher Wanjek *Bad Medicine: Misconceptions and Misuses Revealed, From Distance Healing to Vitamin O.* New York: John Wiley & Sons, 2003.

Andrew Weil *Health and Healing: The Philosophy of Integrative Medicine.* Boston: Houghton Mifflin, 2004.

James C. Whorton	*Nature Cures: The History of Alternative Medicine in America.* New York: Oxford University Press, 2002.
Leonard A. Wisneski and Lucy Anderson	*The Scientific Basis of Integrative Medicine.* Boca Raton, FL: CRC, 2005.

Index